MANUAL OF CAR

CW00569538

Already published

Paediatric Gastroenterology *J.H. Tripp and D.C.A. Candy*
Renal Disease *C.B. Brown*
Clinical Blood Transfusion *M. Brozovic and B. Brozovic*
Haematology *A.S.J. Baughan, A.S.B. Hughes, K.G. Patterson and L. Stirling*
Chest Medicine *J.E. Stark, J.M. Shneerson, C.D.R. Flower and T. Higenbottam*
Gynaecology *T. Varma*
Rheumatology *J.M.H. Moll*

Forthcoming volumes in the Manuals series

Gastroenterology *B.T. Cooper and R.E. Barry*
Infectious Diseases *J.A. Innes*
Neonatal Intensive Care *A.R. Wilkinson*

MANUAL OF CARDIOLOGY

Keith D. Dawkins BSc MD MRCP

Consultant Cardiologist,
Wessex Regional Cardiothoracic Unit,
Southampton General Hospital,
Southampton, UK

Churchill Livingstone

EDINBURGH LONDON MELBOURNE AND NEW YORK 1987

CHURCHILL LIVINGSTONE
Medical Division of Longman Group UK Limited

Distributed in the United States of America by Churchill Livingstone Inc., 1560 Broadway, New York, N.Y. 10036, and by associated companies, branches and representatives throughout the world.

© Longman Group UK 1987 Limited

First published 1987

ISBN 0-443-03147-9

British Library Cataloguing in Publication Data
Dawkins, Keith D.
  Manual of cardiology.
  1. Cardiology
  I. Title
  616.1′2   RC681

Library of Congress Cataloging in Publication Data
Dawkins, Keith D.
  Manual of cardiology.
  (Manuals)
    1. Heart—Diseases—Handbooks, manuals, etc.
2. Cardiology—Handbooks, manuals, etc. I. Title.
[DNLM: 1. Heart Diseases. WG 200 D271m]
RC681.D38 1986   616.1′2   86–11289
ISBN 0–443–03147–9

Produced by Longman Singapore Publishers (Pte) Ltd.
Printed in Singapore.

PREFACE

This book aims to be a practical guide for students and junior medical staff with an interest in cardiology. The format of the book is intentionally didactic and represents the opinions of the author, rather than being an exhaustive review of the subject.

District General Hospitals are appointing increasing numbers of cardiovascular physicians who have access to most types of cardiological investigation including echocardiography, exercise stress testing and ECG monitoring. A close relationship between the District General Hospital and the Regional Centre is vital; one of the aims of this book is to provide a guide for those training in the periphery as to when referral to the Regional Centre is appropriate, either for further investigation or definitive treatment.

Any errors, misconceptions or omissions are the responsibility of the author.

Southampton 1987   K.D.D.

ACKNOWLEDGEMENTS

I would like to thank my many friends and colleagues at the Brompton and St George's hospitals and Stanford University Medical Center who provided thoughts and encouragement during the writing of this book. I am especially indebted to Michael Fowler who critically read much of the manuscript.

To Bente, Sam and Leo

CONTENTS

1. CORONARY ARTERY DISEASE

EPIDEMIOLOGY

Coronary artery disease (CAD) is the most important cause of premature death in the United Kingdom. In the age range 45–54 years, 40% of male deaths and 10% of female deaths are due to CAD, and in the 35–44 age group, deaths from CAD account for 30 and 7% of the male and female deaths respectively.

Data from Canada and the USA show a striking 25% reduction in mortality from CAD since 1965; it is not clear how much of this improvement reflects a reduction due to primary prevention and how much is due to a reduction in the severity or case-fatality rate of the disease. Over a similar period the US diet has been modified such that the intake of milk, cream, butter, eggs and animal fats has been reduced and there has been an increase in consumption of vegetable fats, but these dietary changes have been slow to occur in the UK. Although the improvement in CAD mortality in the UK has not paralleled the dramatic changes in the US, there has been a downward trend since 1979.

In the UK the annual incidence of angina pectoris in middle-aged men is approximately 0.5%, with an overall incidence in men twice that of women. The UK prevalence of angina in men increases from 3–4% in the 40–49 age group to 6–7% in the 60–64 age group. In the year 1978–1979, coronary artery disease accounted for approximately 24 million days lost from work by men in the UK, which represents over 8% of all certified incapacity in men. Cardiovascular disease accounts for 150 000 hospital admissions per annum occupying 7500 beds at any one time.

RISK FACTORS

1. *Lipids and diet*
   An increase in total cholesterol is associated with a higher risk of CAD, furthermore the ratio of risk between patients in the top quintile and the lowest two quintiles of total

1

cholesterol is 2.4. Cholesterol is transported in the blood in the form of lipoproteins, 75% as low density lipoprotein (LDL) and 20% as high density lipoprotien (HDL). An increase in LDL is associated with an increase in CAD, and an inverse relationship exists between CAD and the level of HDL. Alcohol and exercise increase HDL levels. Classification of hyperlipidaemia according to lipoprotein type (Fredrickson) is given in Table 1.1. Serum cholesterol is broadly related to the amount and proportion of fat in the diet; furthermore, polyunsaturated fats have a cholesterol lowering effect.

2. *Smoking*

A linear increase in risk is associated with smoking cigarettes (mortality ratio 2.5 for 20 cigarettes daily). Smoking is linked with personality and social class. Possible mechanisms of toxicity include changes in platelet aggregation, vessel permeability, HDL levels, catecholamine activity and carboxyhaemoglobin formation.

3. *Obesity*

When obesity occurs in isolation (without diabetes mellitus, lipid abnormalities etc.) it is not an important risk factor for CAD.

4. *Diabetes mellitus*

Diabetic men have a 50% higher risk of CAD, and the disease occurs at a younger age in this group. Diabetes mellitus is also associated with obesity, systemic hypertension and Type IV hyperlipidaemia.

5. *Systemic hypertension*

An increase in systemic blood pressure is related to an increase in the incidence of CAD particularly in those over the age of 55 years.

6. *Gender and sex hormones*

At all ages, females have a lower incidence of CAD than men but the rate increases after the menopause. Relative risk of myocardial infarction among oral contraceptive users is 3.5.

7. *Family history*

A higher than expected risk of CAD in first degree relatives is independent of cholesterol, systemic hypertension or smoking history, suggesting a familial predisposition or genetic influence.

8. *Race*

When other risk factors are excluded, Caucasians have a higher incidence of CAD than non-Caucasians.

9. *Geography*

Regional differences in the incidence of CAD are related to

Table 1.1 Classification of hyperlipidaemia (Fredrickson)

Type	Lipoprotein abnormality	Cholesterol	Triglyceride	Treatment*
1. Primary hyperlipidaemia				
I	Chylomicrons	+	+++	Medium chain triglycerides
IIa	LDL (beta)	++	–	Cholestyramine (colestipol, probucol, nicotinic acid)
IIb	LDL (beta) + VLDL (pre-beta)	++	++	Clofibrate or Bezafibrate (cholestyramine, nicotinic acid)
III	'Broad' or 'Floating' beta	++	++	Clofibrate or Bezafibrate
IV	VLDL (pre-beta)	+/–	++	Clofibrate orBezafibrate (nicotinic acid)
V	Chylomicrons + VLDL (pre-beta)	+	++	Clofibrate or Bezafibrate (nicotinic acid)
2. Secondary hyperlipidaemia				
Hypothyroidism	Primary biliary cirrhosis			
Nephrotic syndrome	Oestrogens (including contraceptive pill)			
Diabetes mellitus	Beta adrenergic blockade (beta$_1$)			
Alcohol excess	Thiazide diuretics			

* Prior to drug treatment, all patients should undergo dietary modification (correct obesity, dietary fat to provide <30% total calories, polyunsaturated:saturated ratio 1, <300 mg cholesterol daily). Reduce alcohol intake (IIB, IV), and carbohydrate intake (IV)

many factors including urban living, water hardness and diet.

10. *Social class*

    Lower income groups (Class IV & V) have a higher incidence of CAD in all age groups. Class differences are most marked in women, possibly reflecting smoking habits.

11. *Personality*

    Coronary prone behaviour (Type A personality) has not been shown to be associated with atherosclerosis, but it may lead to myocardial ischaemia (e.g. via coronary artery spasm).

12. *Physical activity*

    A close relationship between activity and personality makes independent assessment of these two risk factors difficult. Exercise increases HDL (see p. 2).

13. *Clotting*

    Increased levels of factor VIII, fibrinogen and blood viscosity are associated with CAD; these changes in the clotting profile may account for the increase in CAD in post-menopausal women.

PATHOPHYSIOLOGY

The simplistic view of angina pectoris as the clinical manifestation of an inbalance between myocardial oxygen supply and demand is being modified by the appreciation that the epicardial coronary artery is a dynamic structure capable of responding to a variety of neural and humoral stimuli.

Fixed obstruction

Fixed anatomical obstruction to coronary arterial flow is caused by atherosclerosis. Resting flow is not affected until there is a 70% reduction in the arterial lumen, although less severe lesions may impair the normal response to an increase in myocardial oxygen demand. Coronary stenoses cause a reduction in myocardial perfusion pressure and ultimately lead to a further discrepancy between oxygen supply and demand due to the elevation in LVEDP and subendocardial ischaemia secondary to impaired left ventricular function.

Coronary vasoreactivity (spasm)

Alterations in vascular tone probably account for much of the variation in 'angina threshold' between one patient and another. Stimuli such as hypoxia and endogenous catecholamine release, as well as the liberation of other vasoactive substances (e.g. serotonin, thromboxane A_2, leukotrienes) determine coronary flow. Furthermore, physical stimuli, for example turbulence within coronary vessels, may lead to an interaction between fixed and dynamic obstruction thus dictating overall coronary flow.

CLINICAL SYNDROMES

1. *Stable angina pectoris*
   A clinical diagnosis of chest pain predictably precipitated by a number of stimuli (see below) and relieved by rest. Abnormalities of the ECG may occur in association with symptoms.

2. *Unstable angina*
   A term that should be limited to angina of increasing severity, also occurring at rest, but stopping short of acute myocardial infarction. The history of unstable angina is usually short (<4 weeks). In the subgroup of patients refractory to intensive medical treatment the chances of progress to myocardial infarction are high.

3. *Variant (Prinzmetal) angina*
   A syndrome of typical angina pectoris, often occurring at rest and associated with transient ST segment elevation on the ECG; this clinical presentation suggests that angina is precipitated by a transient reduction in coronary flow, rather than an increase in myocardial oxygen demand. In some patients the coronary arteries are normal, in others coronary artery spasm can be provoked, and in others ST elevation occurs in the setting of atherosclerotic coronary disease. In view of the heterogeneity of these groups of patients, the term variant angina should probably be dropped.

4. *Angina with normal coronary arteries*
   More common in women, the character of the chest pain may not be typical or exercise related. Some patients may have coronary artery spasm but in the majority no abnormality can be found. Prognosis is excellent although the symptoms can be refractory to medical treatment.

CLINICAL HISTORY

In no condition is an accurate clinical history more important than in angina pectoris. The diagnosis of angina is a clinical diagnosis, and although often accompanied by characteristic changes on the resting or exercise electrocardiogram, exercise thallium scan or coronary arteriogram, a few patients do have typical angina with no detectable abnormalities during investigation.

In the majority of patients, angina can be diagnosed with certainty following a careful clinical history; in a few, doubt will remain because the nature or the localisation of the pain or the relationship to activity will not be typical. In taking the history it is as important to watch the patient for 'non-verbal' clues as to listen to the description of the symptoms.

A number of characteristics of the pain are helpful in making the correct diagnosis:

1. *Localisation*

   Chest pain is situated in the mid sternal region but may be maximal anywhere from the epigastrium to the jaw. Less commonly, the pain may be limited to a more distant site (e.g. left hand, wrist). Left-sided chest pain is not a feature of ischaemic heart disease. In more than 95% of patients pain occurs in the chest and in approximately two thirds of patients the pain radiates (in reducing frequency) to the left arm and wrist, neck, back, right arm and wrist, and lower jaw. Pain radiating to the left arm tends to pass down the inside of the arm to the fourth and fifth fingers, whereas musculoskeletal pain tends to radiate down the lateral aspect of the arm.

2. *Character*

   Well-localised pain is not a feature of angina pectoris. The pain is diffuse and may be illustrated by a clenched fist or the flat of the hand indicating a pressure on the chest rather than by a pointing finger. Descriptive terms used to characterise the pain include ache, pressure, tightness, heaviness and constriction. Burning, stabbing and sharp, implying a more superficial pain are not typical of ischaemic cardiac pain.

3. *Duration*

   Anginal pain is short-lived, often because the patient takes steps to avoid the precipitating factor, or alternatively relieves the attack with self-administered nitrates. Typical attacks last 2–20 minutes, a more prolonged episode may suggest acute myocardial infarction.

4. *Associated symptoms*

   Apprehension, sweating and breathlessness may all occur in association with angina. Occasionally, breathlessness in the absence of chest pain may be the only manifestation of angina, probably due to an elevation in LVEDP and a transient reduction in pulmonary compliance. Pain in the upper limbs may be associated with numbness or tingling in the arm or fingers. Although dizziness may occur with angina, actual syncope is rare.

5. *Precipitating factors*

Exertion (e.g. walking) further exacerbated by the cold or wind. Changes in environment (e.g. leaving a warm room). Anxiety and emotion (including watching television). Isometric stress (e.g. lifting), bending down, or exertion with the arms raised (e.g. shaving, brushing teeth) may all precipitate angina. Smoking is a particularly potent stimulant, and the increased cardiac output required for digestion may provoke post-prandial angina. Angina may occur in bed at night (e.g. during sexual intercourse) or during REM sleep or in association with dreaming.

6. *Relieving factors*

Pain precipitated by exercise is usually promptly relieved by rest. The response to sublingual nitrates is further confirmation of the diagnosis of angina pectoris. In 75% of patients sublingual nitrates relieve symptoms within three minutes; an undue delay in symptomatic relief suggests that the pain is not cardiac, or the GTN tablets are time-expired. Occasional patients can 'walk through' their pain such that the eventual level of exertion achieved is greater than that which initially precipitated the angina. Other activities that may relieve angina include carotid sinus pressure, breath holding and a Valsalva manoeuvre.

PHYSICAL SIGNS

1. *None*

Physical examination in the patient with angina is often unrewarding unless the symptoms have been precipitated by a cause other than coronary artery disease (Table 1.2). The majority of patients have no abnormal physical signs.

Table 1.2

Diseases associated with angina pectoris
1. Coronary artery disease (fixed or dynamic)
2. Aortic stenosis
3. Aortic regurgitation
4. Mitral stenosis
5. Hypertrophic cardiomyopathy
6. Primary pulmonary hypertension

Factors exacerbating angina pectoris
1. Hyperthyroidism
2. Anaemia

2. *Hyperlipidaemia*

   An arcus senilis in patients over 40 years of age need not reflect hyperlipidaemia, but in younger patients the finding may be significant. Similarly, xanthelasma are often seen in patients with normal lipid levels. Tuberous, tendinous and eruptive xanthomas should be sought on the elbows, knees, Achilles tendon, dorsum of the hand and elsewhere, as they are indicative of hyperlipidaemia (see Table 1.1.).

3. *Systemic blood pressure*

   Systemic hypertension is an important risk factor in CAD (see p. 2).

4. *Pulse*

   Assuming the angina is secondary to CAD, the character of the pulse is usually normal. A transient tachycardia accompanies the acute attack, and a resting tachycardia between attacks suggests significant myocardial damage often as the result of a previous myocardial infarction. Occasionally, angina may be precipitated by a tachyarrhythmia (e.g. ventricular tachycardia) which may be apparent on physical examination during the acute attack. Pulsus alternans indicates severe myocardial impairment.

5. *Venous pressure*

   In uncomplicated angina the venous pulse is normal. An elevation in venous pressure suggests previous myocardial infarction (see Ch. 2)

6. *Precordial palpation*

   Complications of CAD (e.g. acute myocardial infarction, LV aneurysm) may provide characteristic abnormalities of the precordial impulse (see Ch. 2), and occasionally a pre-systolic bulge may be palpable due to an increase in left atrial pressure secondary to a reduction in LV compliance.

7. *Auscultation*

   Between attacks of angina, auscultation of the heart is frequently normal. During an attack the reduction in myocardial compliance causes an increase in the left atrial pressure accompanied by an audible S4. Similarly, paradoxical (reversed) splitting of S2 may appear as the clinical manifestation of prolonged left ventricular ejection. An S3 is unusual in angina pectoris unless there is pre-existing myocardial damage. Papillary muscle ischaemia or abnormalities of papillary muscle alignment may result in mild mitral regurgitation characterised by an intermittent late systolic murmur. Of rare interest is the mid-diastolic murmur audible between the left sternal edge and apex from a proximal coronary artery stenosis.

DIFFERENTIAL DIAGNOSIS

If sufficient care is taken to elicit an accurate clinical history, there is little difficulty in deciding on the diagnosis of angina with a high degree of accuracy in the majority of patients. A combination of chest pain radiating to the left arm, precipitated by exertion, relieved by GTN in <3 min and associated with an S4 has a sensitivity of 62% and a specificity of 100% in the diagnosis of organic CAD.

Chest wall and musculoskeletal pain can be differentiated on the clinical history. Gastrointestinal symptoms (e.g. oesophageal spasm, reflux oesophagitis, and peptic ulceration) can usually be differentiated by the association with certain foodstuffs and relief by antacids. Oesophageal spasm may cause difficulty because the pain can be relieved by sublingual GTN and may be associated with non-specific repolarisation changes on the ECG.

INVESTIGATIONS

1. *Electrocardiogram*
   The resting ECG is often unhelpful in the assessment of angina pectoris unless it is recorded during an acute attack. Although there may be evidence of previous myocardial infarction, or changes compatible with an LV aneurysm, approximately 50% of patients have a normal ECG when they are not in pain. Thus, the sensitivity of the resting ECG in detecting CAD (when compared with coronary arteriography) is 50% and the specificity is approximately 70%. In an individual patient it is most helpful to witness changes from the baseline occurring with chest pain.

   Changes in the T wave (e.g. flattening, inversion and tall T waves) are non-specific and may be seen in ventricular hypertrophy, myocarditis, pericarditis, cardiomyopathy and electrolyte disturbance. Reversible changes in the T waves occurring with pain are more suggestive of ischaemia.

   Downsloping ST-segment depression is also non-specific unless occurring with pain; reversible horizontal ST-segment depression is more characteristic of myocardial ischaemia. 'Fixed' ST-segment depression suggests non-Q wave infarction.

2. *Chest radiograph*
   In uncomplicated angina pectoris the chest radiograph is normal. Previous myocardial infarction may give rise to cardiac enlargement or elevation of the pulmonary venous pressure. Occasionally a ventricular aneurysm results in the

characteristic bulge or calcification of the left heart border but these radiographic findings are unreliable.

3. *Exercise testing*

A formal exercise test can be viewed as a natural extension to the clinical examination and ideally should be carried out by the physician who records the clinical history. A number of parameters can be evaluated using an objective exercise test in addition to changes occurring on the ECG (see Table 1.3); furthermore, the results of exercise testing can be used to stratify patients according to prognosis.

A detailed discussion of the various protocols used in exercise testing is beyond the scope of this book. Any protocol used for cardiac exercise testing should be simple, short, reproducible and applicable to a wide range of patients, thus allowing direct comparisons to be made between different patient populations. Both the sensitivity and specificity of exercise testing as a means of identifying patients with CAD can be increased by using a maximal symptom limited test rather than a submaximal or steady-state protocol which is more suitable for the evaluation of other conditions (e.g. pulmonary disease). In practice, most centres now use a standard or modified Bruce protocol (Table 1.4). Exercise testing should only be carried out under medical supervision in an area equipped with adequate facilities for resuscitation (see Ch. 20).

Table 1.3 Data obtained from a formal exercise test

1. Assessment of objective exercise tolerance
2. Nature of symptoms limiting exercise (chest pain, fatigue, breathlessness etc.)
3. Evaluation of haemodynamic response to exercise
4. Document ST segment changes occurring with exercise and during the recovery period
5. Evaluation of exercise induced arrhythmias
6. Document beneficial effects of surgical procedures or medical therapy
7. Risk stratification following acute myocardial infarction
8. Guide to rehabilitation following acute myocardial infarction

Table 1.4 Standard Bruce treadmill exercise protocol

Stage	Speed (mph)	Gradient (%)	Duration (min)
I	1.7	10	3
II	2.5	12	3
III	3.4	14	3
IV	4.2	16	3
V	5.0	18	3
VI	5.5	20	3
VII	6.0	22	3

Blood pressure, pulse rate and 12 lead ECG recorded at rest, and every 3 min until peak exercise, and during recovery every 1 min for 5 min or until the ECG has returned to baseline. Stage 0 (1.7 mph, gradient 0%) may be added for sick, frail or elderly patients.

Physical exercise results in an increase in myocardial oxygen requirement (MVO_2) which is a potent stimulator of angina pectoris in patients with significant CAD. During dynamic exercise (e.g. walking, running) increasing MVO_2 is linearly related to cardiac output, which is mainly brought about by an increase in heart rate. Both systolic and diastolic blood pressure increase with exercise, although the increase in systolic blood pressure is more marked. The 'double product' (peak heart rate × peak systolic blood pressure) correlates well with peak MVO_2.

In patients with CAD, myocardial ischaemia is reflected as ST segment depression. Assuming a 12 lead ECG system is used, ST segment changes are seen most commonly in the lead with the tallest R wave (usually V_5). In 10% of patients, ST changes are limited to the inferior leads. Thus, with a three channel machine recording leads I, aVF and V_5 will identify most ECG changes occurring with exercise. Reasons for terminating the exercise test are listed in Table 1.5.

Criteria for 'significant' ST segment depression represent a compromise between sensitivity and specificity (Fig. 1.1 and Table 1.6). Most series define significant ST depression as being 1 mm or more planar or down-sloping depression 80 ms

Table 1.5 Reasons for terminating an exercise test

1. Symptomatic (angina, breathlessness, exhaustion etc.)
2. Fall in systemic blood pressure
3. Peripheral circulatory insufficiency
4. Sustained arrhythmias (e.g. VT)
5. Heart block
6. Failure of ECG apparatus
7. Diagnostic ST shift
8. Target heart rate or grade of exercise achieved

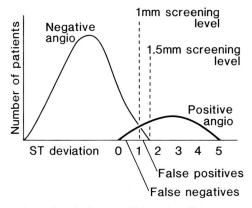

Fig. 1.1 Influence of screening criteria on sensitivity and specificity

Table 1.6 Terms used in exercise testing

Sensitivity: $\dfrac{\text{True positives detected}}{\text{Total number true positives}}$

Specificity: $\dfrac{\text{True negatives (normals) detected}}{\text{Total number of normals}}$

Predictive accuracy: $\dfrac{\text{Number of true tests (true positives + true negatives)}}{\text{Total number of tests}}$

Predictive value: $\dfrac{\text{True positives}}{\text{True positives + false positives}}$

Bayes' theorem: Predictive value of a test not only depends on the sensitivity, but also the prevalence of the disease in the population being tested

after the J point. Other patterns of ST segment shift include J point depression (a normal accompaniment of tachycardia), upsloping depression and ST elevation. An increase in R wave amplitude may accompany myocardial ischaemia although the mechanism remains unclear.

4. *Myocardial scintigraphy*

Radionuclide imaging is not usually necessary as part of the routine investigation of patients with angina. In certain patients (e.g. with LBBB) where interpretation of the exercise ECG is impossible, myocardial scintigraphy may assist in the accurate diagnosis of CAD. Although the technique will frequently identify the area of the myocardium involved, coronary arteriography is still required to accurately delineate coronary anatomy prior to coronary artery bypass grafting.

Two radionuclides are in widespread clinical use, ^{201}thallium and ^{99m}technetium.

Uptake of ^{201}thallium is proportional to myocardial perfusion and is relatively homogeneous throughout the ventricular mass. For the detection of CAD, ^{201}thallium imaging is combined with a symptom limited maximal exercise test (either treadmill or bicycle). Thallium (1.5–2.0 mCi) is injected into a peripheral vein at peak exercise, and images obtained on a gamma scintillation counter 5–10 minutes later demonstrate regional myocardial perfusion at peak exercise. In order to differentiate myocardial scars or previous myocardial infarction, a further set of images are recorded 2.5–3.0 hours after exercise to determine whether the defects are 'fixed' or there is evidence of 'redistribution' suggestive of reversible ischaemia. The sensitivity and specificity of exercise ^{201}thallium imaging for the detection of CAD is 83% and 90% respectively.

Global and segmental ventricular function can be assessed by gated blood pool scanning using ^{99m}Tc-pertechnetate

(MUGA). Labelled albumin or autologous red cells are injected into a peripheral vein and a gated blood pool image obtained at rest in order to derive the resting ejection fraction. Symptom limited supine bicycle exercise is then undertaken and the exercise ejection fraction calculated together with any segmental wall motion abnormality provoked by exercise. A failure to increase the ejection fraction by 5% or more in association with a new exercise induced regional wall abnormality has a sensitivity of 86% and a specificity of 91% for CAD.

5. *M-mode and cross-sectional echocardiography*
   M-mode echocardiography has little value in the routine assessment of patients with angina pectoris. The cross-sectional technique may reveal regional wall abnormalities, myocardial scars or an LV aneurysm, but the study may be entirely normal in stable angina.

6. *Coronary arteriography*
   Cardiac catheterisation is appropriate for certain subgroups of patients (see Ch. 3).

MEDICAL MANAGEMENT

General measures

1. *Smoking*
   The risk of subsequent myocardial infarction is reduced by 50% 5 years after stopping smoking. Relative risk (compared with non-smokers) returns to normal 10 years after stopping smoking.

2. *Diet*
   In general, the evidence that alterations in diet can favourably affect the incidence of symptomatic CAD is unimpressive. In certain subgroups (e.g. familial hyperlipidaemia; see Table 1.1), modification of the lipid profile by diet or drugs appears to be worthwhile, but in the vast majority of patients with elevation of serum cholesterol and/or triglycerides the results of available trials are inconclusive.

   Common sense would indicate that the avoidance of obesity is important, although given that many patients who give up smoking subsequently put on weight, ceasing smoking is far more significant than any associated increase in weight. In general, cholesterol intake should be reduced and only 25–30% calories taken in the form of fat. Vegetable oils are substituted for animal fats such that saturated and unsaturated fats are taken in equal proportion. Currently, drug therapy cannot be recommended in the treatment of the more common types of hyperlipidaemia. Similarly, the results of multiple risk factor intervention trials have been disappointing.

3. *Exercise*

Conclusive data showing a beneficial effect of exercise on the incidence of CAD are lacking. However, a regular exercise programme is likely to be associated with a more healthy lifestyle in general (diet, non-smoker etc.) and there appears to be a lower incidence of CAD in fit, healthy patients. Once CAD is manifest there are no good data to indicate that exercise reduces the risk of a further cardiac event. In particular, sudden unaccustomed exercise in the patient with CAD may be catastrophic.

Specific therapy

Nitrates

Nitrates act as systemic venodilators causing a reduction in 'preload' by pooling blood in the venous capacitance vessels; in addition they act as direct coronary vasodilators. The reduction in 'preload' results in an increase in coronary perfusion pressure which relieves subendocardial ischaemia. Furthermore, coronary artery spasm can be inhibited by nitrates. The action of the nitrates at the cellular level is ill understood. Nitrate preparations are listed in Table 1.7.

1. *Sublingual nitrates*

Sublingual nitrates remain one of the most valuable forms of therapy in angina pectoris. All too often inadequate instruction is given to the patient regarding the appropriate use of this drug. Sublingual administration has the advantage of a rapid onset of action with peak blood levels at 2 minutes and a plasma half-life of 7 minutes; the sublingual route avoids the extensive first pass hepatic metabolism occurring with other oral nitrates. 75% of patients obtain symptomatic relief within 3 minutes and a further 15% within 15 minutes of administration. Sublingual nitrates (glyceryl trinitrate 0.5 mg) should be used liberally, with an explanation to the patient that the drug is not addictive, nor will tolerance develop with prolonged usage. GTN should also be taken on a prophylactic basis, in anticipation of indulging in activity likely to provoke chest pain, used in this way the beneficial effects may last for up to one hour. Side effects include headache, cutaneous flushing, postural dizziness and reflex tachycardia. Side effects can be minimised by taking the drug whilst sitting, and removing the partially dissolved tablet from

Table 1.7 Nitrate preparations available in the UK

Nitroglycerin	
Intravenous	Nitrocine
Glyceryl trinitrate	
Sublingual	GTN (0.3, 0.5, 0.6 mg)
Buccal	Suscard Buccal (1, 2, 3, 5 mg)
Aerosol	Cor-Nitro (0.4 mg), Nitrolingual (0.4 mg),
Sustained release	Nitrocontin Continus (2.6, 6.4 mg),
	Sustac (2.6, 6.4 mg)
Percutaneous	Percutol (2%), Transiderm-Nitro (25,50 mg)
Intravenous	Tridil
Isosorbide mononitrate	
Oral	Elantan (20, 40 mg), Ismo 20 (20 mg),
	Monit (20 mg), Mono-Cedocard (20, 40 mg)
Isosorbide dinitrate	
Oral	Cedocard (5, 10, 20 mg), Isoket (5, 10, 20 mg),
	Isordil (5, 20, 30 mg), Sorbitrate (10, 20 mg),
	Vascardin (10, 30 mg)
Sublingual	Isordil SL (5 mg), Sorbichew (5 mg),
Sustained release	Cedocard Retard (20 mg), Isoket Retard (20 mg),
	Isordil Tembids (40 mg), Soni-Slo (20, 40 mg),
	Sorbid SA (40 mg)
Intravenous	Cedocard, Isoket
Pentaerythritol tetranitrate	
Oral	Peritrate (10 mg), Cardiacap (30 mg),
	Mycardol (30 mg)
Sustained release	Peritrate SA (80 mg)

the mouth once the angina has been relieved. Chewing the tablet may expedite the onset of action.

GTN tablets are volatile and have a shelf life of 2–3 months. If they are stored in a dark bottle in the refrigerator and without any packing material (e.g. cotton wool) they remain effective for 6 months. An alternative but more costly preparation is Nitrolingual spray which gives a metered dose of 0.4 mg GTN per application with a shelf life in excess of 3 years.

2. *Long-acting oral nitrates*
Oral nitrates undergo extensive first-pass hepatic metabolism and degradation into inactive metabolites. Dinitrates are transformed into two mononitrates which are bioactive and have a prolonged duration of action. It is likely that the beneficial effects of the dinitrates are due to these active metabolites in addition to the eventual saturation of the hepatic enzymes. More recently, isosorbide mononitrate has become available which has the advantage of virtually complete bioavailability without the disadvantage of first-pass metabolism. The onset of pharmacological action occurs within 20 minutes, and therapeutic blood levels can be maintained for 8 hours on a twice or thrice daily regimen starting at a dose of 20 mg twice daily. Tolerance may occur

but is rarely a problem in clinical practice. Other long-acting nitrates include buccal and chewable preparations.

3. *Transcutaneous nitrates*

   Topical nitrate preparations offer a satisfactory alternative to long-acting oral nitrates. Skin absorption is rapid, although variable, and avoids first-pass hepatic metabolism. They may be particularly useful in the control of nocturnal symptoms. GTN ointment or paste (Percutol) is messy to apply, but one of the newer patch delivery systems (e.g. Transiderm) may be more acceptable with a significant blood level obtained within two hours and lasting in excess of 24 hours. Skin sensitivity remains a problem and the transcutaneous nitrates are expensive.

4. *Intravenous nitrates*

   Intravenous nitrates are now used routinely in the management of unstable angina and in patients requiring vasodilator therapy (see Ch. 7). In clinical practice there is little to choose between preparations of isosorbide (e.g. Cedocard, Isoket, Isordil) or nitroglycerin (Nitrocine). PVC administration sets should be avoided as up to 40% of the activity of the nitrate may be lost. Dose requirements vary dramatically, and the usual approach is to increase the infusion progressively until systemic hypotension (systolic BP <100 mmHg) occurs. Control of angina is usual within the dose range 2–15 mg/h isosorbide or 10–400 mcg/min nitroglycerine. Side effects are similar to oral nitrates.

Beta blockade

Beta adrenergic blocking drugs continue to be the mainstay of the drug treatment of angina pectoris. Beta blockers are competitive inhibitors of catecholamine binding at beta receptor sites and reduce the myocardial oxygen requirements (MVO_2) by two routes; firstly, a direct myocardial action reduces LV systolic pressure and the rate of pressure rise (dp/dt), and secondly the 'double-product' (heart rate × systolic arterial pressure) is reduced in response to exercise; thus, 'afterload' is reduced as a result of a reduction in aortic impedance. The net effect of beta blockers on coronary blood flow is controversial; a reduction in heart rate leads to an improvement in (diastolic) coronary perfusion, but the unopposed alpha action on coronary vessels may be deleterious.

At the present time nine beta blockers can be prescribed in the United Kingdom (Table 1.8), and it is likely that more will become available in the future. Three factors are important in choosing the appropriate beta blocker; namely, cardio-selectivity, frequency of dosing, and patient acceptability. Drug manufacturers make much of the other differences in the secondary properties of individual agents (e.g. partial agonist activity, membrane stabilising activity and local anaesthetic action), but in clinical practice these are of little importance.

Table 1.8 Characteristics of the available beta blockers

Drug	B₁ selectivity	Absorption (%)	Bioavailability (%)	Protein binding (%)	Lipophilic	Plasma half-life	Dose range (mg/day)
Propranolol	−	>90	30	93	++	3–6 h	60–480
Oxprenolol	−				+	1–3 h	60–480
Nadolol	−	30	30	30	−	14–24 h	40–240
Acebutolol	−/+				+	3 h	400–1200
Sotalol	−				−	15–18 h	160–600
Timolol	−	>90	75	10	+	3–6 h	10–60
Metoprolol	+	>95	50	12	+	2–4 h	100–400
Atenolol	+	50	40	<5	−	6–9 h	50–200
Pindolol	+	>90	90	57	+	3–4 h	10–45

1. *Cardio-selectivity*

   Beta receptors can be sub-divided into beta$_1$ and beta$_2$ receptors. Beta$_1$ receptors when stimulated increase the rate and force of cardiac contraction, increase renin release and increase the release of free fatty acids; whereas beta$_2$ stimulation causes bronchodilatation, arteriolar dilatation, hepatic gluconeogenesis, insulin release and relaxation of the pregnant uterus. It must be emphasized that the beta receptor population is not static and may be altered by disease, age and drug status; furthermore, cardio-selectivity is dose related, the degree of 'selectivity' varying from patient to patient. Preparations that preferentially block beta$_1$ activity (e.g. Atenolol, Metoprolol) may be better tolerated than non-selective agents (see p. 17), but in certain conditions (e.g. hypertrophic cardiomyopathy) a non-selective preparation (e.g. Propranolol) may be more appropriate (see Ch. 6).

2. *Frequency of dosing*

   Unfortunately there is little relationship between the oral dose, plasma level and the duration of the pharmacological effect of particular beta blocking drugs. Possible factors responsible for individual variation include variable first-pass hepatic metabolism and plasma drug binding, production of active metabolites, variable concentrations of the active ($-$) isomer and differences in the 'sympathetic tone' between individuals. In most patients control of angina is adequate on a once daily regimen (e.g. Propranolol LA 160 mg daily or Atenolol 100 mg daily), although in some individuals 'break-through' angina occurs in the evening, in which case an additional dose may be required in the late afternoon. In 20–30% of patients with angina there is little symptomatic improvement on beta blockers, possibly due to inadequate dosing or unopposed alpha adrenergic action.

3. *Side-effects*

   Side-effects sufficient to cause withdrawal of the drug occur in 5–10% of patients and are listed in Table 1.9. In general, side-effects are more commonly encountered with non-selective agents and in those with high lipid solubility (because they cross the blood-brain barrier).

4. *Contraindications*

   Beta blockers are contraindicated in patients with severe airflow obstruction, myocardial impairment, high grade atrioventricular block or severe peripheral vascular disease. In many patients however small doses of beta blockers can be introduced under hospital supervision without untoward side-effects.

Table 1.9 Side-effects of beta blocking drugs

Cardiovascular
Low cardiac output, sinus bradycardia, atrioventricular block, systemic hypotension,
?exacerbate coronary artery 'spasm', precipitate myocardial ischaemia following acute
withdrawal. Cool extremities, exacerbate peripheral vascular disease, Raynaud's phenomenon.
Muscle fatigue, reduced exercise tolerance

Pulmonary
Exacerbate airflow obstruction (bronchial asthma, obstructive bronchitis, emphysema)

Gastrointestinal
Anorexia, nausea, diarrhoea

Central nervous system
Depression, insomnia, vivid dreams, hallucinations, impaired concentration, drowsiness,
impotence

Metabolic
Hyperlipidaemia ($\uparrow$ triglyceride, $\uparrow$ VLDL, $\downarrow$ HDL), potentiate hypoglycaemia)

Skin
Rash, oculomucocutaneous syndrome (rash, dry eyes, sclerosing peritonitis)

Calcium antagonists

Under the heading 'calcium antagonists' (or calcium channel blockers)
are a heterogeneous group of drugs that inhibit the slow current channel
by which calcium ions enter the cell and initiate smooth muscle
contraction and intracardiac conduction. Although it is convenient to
consider these drugs as a group, their properties are very different (Table
1.10).

Table 1.10 Properties of the calcium antagonists

	Nifedipine	Verapamil	Diltiazem
Site of action			
Peripheral arterioles	+++	++	++
Coronary arteries	+/−	+	+/−
Conduction tissue	−	+++	++
Efficacy			
Systemic hypertension	+++	++	−
Angina pectoris	+++	+++	+++
'Supraventricular tachycardia'	−	+++	−
Pharmcokinetics			
Dose (8 hourly)	10–20	80–160	60–90
Oral absorption (%)	95	>90	>90
Bioavailability (%)	40–60	10–20	45
Time to onset of action (min)	<20	<30	<30
Protein binding (%)	>90	90	80–90
Plasma elimination half-life (h)	4–5	3–7	4–7
Therapeutic level (ng/ml)	25–100	80–400	50–300
Renal excretion (%)*	85	75	35

* Remainder gastrointestinal

Calcium antagonists reduce 'afterload' by inhibiting contraction of arterial smooth muscle, with little action on the venous capacitance vessels. By a similar mechanism calcium antagonists result in coronary artery vasodilatation and are therefore particularly useful in the treatment of 'vasospastic' angina. Conduction through the atrioventricular node is inhibited and is considered in more detail in Chapter 16. Finally, there is a direct negative inotropic action on cardiac muscle which is demonstrable in isolated muscle preparations but in clinical practice is offset by the benefits of arterial vasodilatation.

Calcium antagonists can be used in the treatment of angina pectoris, systemic hypertension (Ch. 4), hypertrophic cardiomyopathy (Ch. 6) and tachyarrhythmias (Ch. 16).

1. *Verapamil*

   Oral verapamil is an effective anti-anginal agent and like other calcium antagonists is useful in the treatment of patients unable to tolerate beta blocking drugs (e.g. due to bronchial asthma, peripheral vascular disease). It may also be combined with other agents as part of a 'stepped-care' approach to the treatment of angina (see p. 21).

   Peak action of oral verapamil occurs three hours after ingestion, and although absorption is excellent, extensive first-pass hepatic metabolism reduces bioavailability to only 10–20%. Doses of verapamil should be reduced in patients with hepatic disease. Excretion is via the kidneys and gut.

   Early reports on the use of verapamil in angina were disappointing probably due to the low doses used in these studies. When used in the range 120–160 mg three times daily, verapamil is at least as effective as beta blockade in the relief of angina. In these circumstances the primary action of the drug is thought to be on the peripheral arterial smooth muscle, rather than a direct effect on the coronary circulation. Verapamil has been widely used in the treatment of 'variant' angina secondary to coronary artery spasm.

   Side-effects include facial flushing, nausea, dizziness and constipation which may be intolerable when high doses of the drug are used. Conduction disease is a contraindication to the use of verapamil, and if digoxin is used in combination with verapamil the dose of digoxin may need reducing due to a reduction in renal excretion.

2. *Nifedipine*

   Of the various calcium antagonists currently available, nifedipine is the drug of choice for the management of stable or 'variant' angina. It is a powerful arterial vasodilator with little or no action on the conduction system. Unlike verapamil, first-pass hepatic metabolism is not a problem with close to 100% absorption and 40–60% bioavailability. Furthermore, peak plasma levels occur less than one hour after oral ingestion. More rapid absorption can be achieved by breaking or biting a nifedipine capsule and allowing sublingual absorption of the liquid. An oral dose of 10–40 mg three or four daily is usually required for effective treatment, but the recently introduced slow-release preparation may allow twice daily dosing to be adequate. An intravenous preparation will shortly be available in the UK.

Side-effects are similar but more frequent to those seen with verapamil. Ankle swelling occurs in 20–30% of patients and does not respond predictably to diuretics. There are rare reports of angina being provoked by nifedipine, and acute pulmonary oedema can occasionally be precipitated by the drug.

3. *Diltiazem*

Little comparative data are available for the use of diltiazem in angina. Diltiazem shares properties of verapamil and nifedipine being an effective coronary and peripheral arterial vasodilator with additional activity on the conducting system. Usual dose is 30–90 mgs three times daily. Preliminary reports suggest that diltiazem is better tolerated than the other calcium antagonists, although the spectrum of side-effects is similar.

Stepped-care therapy in the treatment of angina pectoris

1. *Stable angina pectoris*

Avoid or treat precipitating factors (e.g. smoking, systemic hypertension). Commence sublingual nitrates to be used on an 'as required' and prophylactic basis. Most patients will require a beta blocker. In 10–20% of patients additional drugs will be needed, either in the form of long-acting nitrates or calcium antagonists. Angina occurring at rest suggests coronary artery 'spasm', in which case calcium antagonists (with or without nitrates) are preferable to beta blockade.

When symptomatic improvement has been achieved, all patients should undergo a formal treadmill exercise test (see p. 10), and coronary arteriography may be considered in certain subgroups of patients (see Ch. 3).

2. *Unstable angina*

In view of the significant risk of early acute myocardial infarction (5–10% within 30 days), patients with unstable angina should be admitted to hospital and treated aggressively. Initially, intravenous nitrates may be necessary to control symptoms, together with oral 'triple therapy' (beta blockade + nitrates + calcium antagonists).

Once acute myocardial infarction has been excluded and the patient rendered asymptomatic, most patients with a history of unstable angina will come to coronary arteriography (see Ch. 3). In occasional patients, maximal medical therapy fails to control the angina; if facilities for intraaortic balloon counter-pulsation are available, this can be very effective and will allow stabilisation of the patient prior to coronary arteriography and urgent myocardial revascularisation.

PROGNOSIS

An accurate estimation of prognosis in individual patients with angina pectoris is difficult, although it is clear that the mortality in medically treated patients is improving with time. Most series quote an annual mortality of 1–10%, determined mostly by the extent of coronary artery disease together with the presence or absence of additional risk factors including diabetes mellitus, systemic hypertension, previous myocardial infarction, obesity, and an abnormal resting electrocardiogram.

2. ACUTE MYOCARDIAL INFARCTION

ERRATUM

Page 23 Line 1
for 150 read 150 000

ㅤn accounts for approximately 150 deaths each ㅤs. There are significant regional differences in ㅤnic heart disease with the highest incidence in ㅤwest in the South-East. Factors implicated in ㅤ rate include smoking habits, gender, ㅤr hardness and climate.

PATHOPHYSIOLOGY

An acute myocardial infarct occurs when myocardial ischaemia is sufficient to cause irreversible necrosis of cardiac muscle. The myocardium is dependent on aerobic metabolism and in normal circumstances myocardial oxygen demands are met by an efficient system of autoregulation in coronary blood flow which may be compromised by fixed (e.g. atherosclerosis) or dynamic (e.g. spasm) coronary artery disease. Major determinants of myocardial oxygen consumption include heart rate, contractility, and systolic wall stress. Wall tension is load dependent, and therefore affected by venous filling ('preload') and peripheral arterial resistance ('afterload'), and inversely proportional to wall thickness.

A number of factors contribute to the development of an acute myocardial infarct:

1. *Coronary thrombosis*

    Acute myocardial infarction is not necessarily synonymous with coronary thrombosis. The incidence of thrombosis is highest in patients dying early after an infarct, suggesting that spontaneous thrombolysis occurs if the patient survives the acute event. When thrombosis is present, it is usually superimposed on an atheromatous plaque, which may have ulcerated or contain haemorrhage (a 'complicated' plaque or plaque-fissure). Thrombosis may occur before an infarct, or as a result of infarction. Some patients dying of an infarct have no evidence of thrombosis, whereas others have thrombosis of a major coronary artery which has not led to necrosis of cardiac muscle.

2. *Coronary artery spasm*

   Approximately 5% of patients dying from myocardial infarction have normal coronary arteries and it is likely that coronary artery spasm is responsible for some of these deaths. Spasm may also be related to organic coronary artery disease (atherosclerosis) and in these circumstances an episode of spasm at the site of an atheromatous plaque, with or without superadded thrombosis, may be sufficient to cause a critical reduction in myocardial perfusion. The assumption that coronary artery spasm plays a major role in the pathogenesis of myocardial infarction forms a rational basis for the use of nitrates and calcium antagonists in coronary artery disease.

3. *Collateral vessels*

   The rate at which coronary artery narrowing develops is important in determining the functional consequences of a particular lesion. When the disease progresses slowly, subsequent occlusion of the vessel may not be associated with haemodynamic compromise due to the development of collateral vessels. These vessels account for the occasional patient who at cardiac catheterisation is shown to have proximal occlusion of all three coronary vessels.

SUBENDOCARDIAL VS TRANSMURAL INFARCTION

The majority of coronary flow occurs in early diastole and uniform transmural blood flow is maintained by coronary autoregulation. When autoregulation is lost (e.g. in coronary atherosclerosis), perfusion of the subendocardial region is particularly susceptible to compromise which may be compounded by vasoconstriction mediated by endogenous catecholamine release. Subendocardial infarction is less likely to result in haemodynamic deterioration, although ventricular arrhythmias and sudden death may complicate even the smallest myocardial infarct. Occlusion of a major coronary vessel causes transmural infarction, involving the full-thickness of the ventricular wall. Consequences of transmural infarction include myocardial rupture, ventricular septal defect, and left ventricular aneurysm. Wide variations in coronary artery anatomy, in particular the dominance of the coronary circulation will affect the area of myocardium in jeopardy. Occlusion of the left anterior descending coronary artery involves the anterior free wall, the apical region of the left ventricle, and parts of the interventricular septum. A left circumflex lesion affects the posterior and inferolateral left ventricular walls, and an occlusion of the right coronary artery causes infarction in the inferior septum, and the inferoposterior region of the left ventricle (an area shared with the left circumflex coronary artery and perfused variably depending on coronary artery dominance).

CLINICAL HISTORY

Up to 50% of patients who sustain a myocardial infarct have a previous history of cardiovascular disease which may include angina, intermittent claudication, transient ischaemic attacks or systemic hypertension.

1. *Chest pain*

   At least 80% of patients present with pain, which is typified by prolonged chest pain indistinguishable in character from angina (see p. 6). Whereas a typical attack of angina lasts 5–10 minutes, and improves with rest or sublingual nitrates, the pain of acute infarction usually lasts at least 30 minutes, despite attempts by the patient to relieve the pain with nitrates. Occasionally the pain may be atypical, for example situated in the epigastrium and radiating to the chest, in which case intraabdominal pathology may be wrongly suspected. Approximately 20% of myocardial infarctions are not associated with pain, particularly in the elderly and those suffering from diabetes mellitus.

   An acute infarct rarely occurs at the time of severe exertion, although it may follow a bout of unusual exertion or emotion in a minority of patients. Up to 50% of patients are awoken form sleep by chest pain and 30% of patients continue with their activities despite the presence of chest pain. Vague symptoms (e.g. general malaise, fatigue, non-specific chest pain) in the few hours or days prior to the acute event occur in approximately half the patients.

2. *Breathlessness*

   Sudden breathlessness related to a sudden rise in left ventricular end diastolic pressure may accompany the chest pain or occur as the sole manifestation of myocardial infarction. Following a silent infarct progressive effort dyspnoea or fatigue may be the only indication of severe left ventricular dysfunction.

3. *Gastrointestinal symptoms*

   Increased vagal activity is responsible for nausea and vomiting which is said to be more common in inferior infarction. In occasional patients the symptoms may be mainly gastrointestinal giving rise to diagnostic confusion between acute infarction and gall bladder disease or peptic ulceration. Diaphragmatic stimulation from an inferior infarct may also cause hiccoughs.

4. *Other symptoms*
These include apprehension, sweating, palpitations, syncope, sudden death (see Ch. 16) and symptoms from an arterial embolism.

PHYSICAL EXAMINATION

1. *General appearance*
Sympathetic overactivity is responsible for the patient appearing pale, sweaty and apprehensive with cool peripheries. A clenched fist held against the precordium may be one of the non-verbal clues alerting the physician to the diagnosis. The patient may be tachypnoeic and prefer to sit up due to an elevated LVEDP. An elevation in LVEDP also provokes a dry cough which may progress in patients with extensive infarction to frank pulmonary oedema with frothy pink sputum. Physical examination should include a search for clinical evidence of hyperlipidaemia. A moderate fever (<38°C) occurs 12–24 hours after an infarct and in association with chest pain is a useful pointer to the diagnosis of myocardial infarction prior to receiving the results of cardiac enzyme estimations.

2. *Pulse and blood pressure*
Sinus tachycardia (100–120/min) occurs in one third of patients. Profound bradycardia or tachycardia may indicate heart block or arrhythmia complicating the infarct. Appropriate analgesia restores a more normal heart rate in most patients unless there is severe ischaemic myocardial damage. Moderate elevation in the blood pressure is attributable to catecholamine release. Hypotension may complicate over-use of nitrates by the patient, or herald the onset of cardiogenic shock (see p. 37). Most patients with a prior history of systemic hypertension have a normal or mildly elevated blood pressure after a myocardial infarct but a hypertensive response is occasionally seen.

3. *Examination of the heart*
Palpation of the precordium may reveal an area of dyskinesis medial to the apex beat, particularly in patients who have sustained an extensive anterior infarct. A presystolic 'a' wave may also be palpable and a sustained apex beat gives a clue to pre-existing systemic hypertension. Acute mitral regurgitation or a ventricular septal defect complicating

myocardial infarction are accompanied by a systolic thrill palpable over the precordium (see p. 39).

The heart sounds may be difficult to hear clearly. A fourth heart sound (S4) is present in virtually all patients although it may be transient. More severe left ventricular dysfunction is associated with a third heart sound (S3) and reversed splitting of the second sound (i.e. delay in A_2 sufficient to allow P_2 to precede A_2, such that splitting of the second sound is maximal on expiration rather than inspiration). Other causes of this finding include LBBB and systemic hypertension. Quiet late systolic murmurs indicate mitral regurgitation secondary to papillary muscle dysfunction or a dilated mitral annulus and come and go depending on loading conditions. Pericardial friction rubs when they occur are often transient and are rarely heard until the second or third day, or much later (up to 6 weeks) as a feature of Dressler's syndrome (see p. 41).

4. *Examination of the lungs*
   End inspiratory crackles are frequently audible over the lung bases even when there is no radiographic evidence of pulmonary oedema. This finding is therefore not necessarily an indication for diuretic therapy. Signs of frank pulmonary oedema are seen in patients following extensive myocardial infarction and wheezing may be prominent in patients with pre-existing airflow obstruction.

5. *Other features*
   Evidence of peripheral vascular disease may be apparent with arterial bruits, absent peripheral pulses and trophic changes in the lower limbs. Examination of the optic fundi should not be omitted as hypertensive and diabetic retinopathy may be evident.

INVESTIGATIONS

Cardiac enzymes

Death of myocardial tissue is associated with liberation of the cytoplasmic constituents of myocardial cells into the circulation. Plots of the time-activity curves of these enzymes (Fig. 2.1) allow the diagnosis of acute myocardial infarction to be made with certainty. Sequential measurements of a panel of cardiac enzymes are more reliable than a single estimation and may accurately time the acute event when this is unclear from the clinical history.

No single enzyme is specific for myocardial infarction, but the more recent use of isoenzymes (e.g. CPK.MB, LDH_1) can improve the

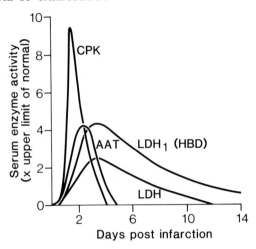

Fig. 2.1 Time-activity curves of cardiac enzymes

specificity of the technique. A two-fold elevation above the upper limit
of the normal range is taken as significant.

1. *Creatine kinase (CPK)*

   This is the first enzyme to appear in the peripheral blood
   initially detected 6–8 hours after the acute event, peaking at
   24 hours and returning to normal within 3 days. CPK may be
   released from skeletal muscle (e.g. from an injection site),
   and increases with pulmonary embolism, alcoholism, diabetes
   mellitus, and following convulsions.

   An isoenzyme of CPK.MB is specific for heart muscle, but
   it can also be released in myocarditis, cardiac trauma
   (including surgery and DC countershock), as well as acute
   myocardial infarction. In some patients CPK.MB may be
   elevated after myocardial infarction when total CPK is
   normal. A failure to detect a significant increase in plasma
   CPK.MB within 18 hours of the onset of chest pain
   effectively excludes an infarct.

2. *Aspartate amino transferase (AAT)*

   Although this enzyme is non-specific it has the advantage that
   it is run as part of the standard biochemical screen in most
   laboratories. AAT can be detected as early as 12 hours and
   peaks at 36 hours. Plasma levels return to normal by 4 days.
   AAT may also be elevated in hepatic congestion (e.g.
   secondary to acute myocardial infarction), primary liver
   disease, pulmonary embolism, and it is a constituent of
   skeletal muscle.

3. *Lactate dehydrogenase (LDH)*

   An elevation in LDH occurs late after myocardial infarction.

Increased activity exceeds the normal range from 24 hours, peaks at 3–6 days and may remain elevated for 2 weeks. LDH is also released in hepatic congestion, primary liver disease, haemolysis, neoplasia and pulmonary embolism. Specificity is increased by measuring the isoenzyme LDH_1 or hydroxybutyrate dehydrogenase (HBD) which can be isolated by electrophoresis. A rise in LDH_1 precedes an increase in total LDH. LDH_1 is also found in red blood cells and may therefore increase with haemolysis.

Serial measurements of cardiac enzymes (e.g. CPK.MB) allow an estimation of infarct size, and provide some information regarding prognosis in a particular patient. Therapeutic manoeuvres designed to limit infarct size can be assessed by monitoring their affect on reducing the amount of enzyme released.

Other blood tests

1. *White cell count*
   Increases from 48 hours in response to myocardial necrosis. Typically 10–15 000 with a polymorphonuclear leucocytosis and a left shift.

2. *Sedimentation rate (ESR)*
   Peaks on day 4 or 5 and may increase again in association with Dressler's syndrome.

3. *Hyperglycaemia*
   Carbohydrate intolerance persisting for some weeks is common in acute myocardial infarction. Patients with previously well controlled diabetes mellitus may become ketoacidotic and are therefore best managed with a continuous infusion of low dose insulin. Both hypoglycemia from over enthusiastic diabetic control and acidosis from inadequate control have an adverse effect on left ventricular function.

4. *Lipids*
   Catecholamine release, recumbency and change in diet which accompany myocardial infarction may affect lipid values. Estimations should therefore be deferred until the first outpatient clinic visit (4 weeks after discharge).

5. *Myoglobin and myosin*
   Myoglobin can be demonstrated in the serum as early as 2 hours after acute infarction. Peak levels occur at approximately 10 hours which is earlier than CPK.MB. However, this test is non-specific as skeletal and myocardial myoglobin are identical. Cardiac myosin appears to be immunologically different from skeletal myosin and this assay offers promise for the future.

Electrocardiography

The combination of a typical clinical history and elevation of the cardiac enzymes is more reliable than the electrocardiogram in the diagnosis of acute myocardial infarction. Electrocardiography has a predictive accuracy of approximately 80% for the diagnosis of acute myocardial infarction, therefore a normal ECG does not exclude recent or previous infarction. However, ECG abnormalities are seen in the majority of patients and if a 'current of injury' is present together with pathological Q waves the likelihood of myocardial infarction is high. Serial ECGs are particularly valuable in documenting the evolution of the electrical disturbances.

The ECG changes of an acute myocardial infarct evolve in a well defined order although the time course will vary from patient to patient.

1. *ST segment shift ('current of injury')*

   Incomplete repolarization of the damaged myocardium causes ST segment elevation as a result of a net flow of current towards the electrodes overlying the affected region. In patients seen very early after infarction, tall, symmetrical T waves may be apparent which become inverted as the ST segments rise. ST segment elevation is convex upwards in the leads facing the infarct and depressed in the leads opposite the infarct (reciprocal depression). T-wave inversion occurs within 24 hours of the acute event and may become more marked ('arrow-head') as the ST segments return to the isoelectric line. The T-waves may remain inverted indefinitely although this finding alone is entirely non-specific.

2. *Q waves*

   ST segment elevation is followed by the development of Q waves. A pathological Q wave is defined as a Q wave of >30 ms duration and >25% the height of the ensuing R wave. Slight broadening of the QRS may be seen very early after infarction and as the Q waves develop there is a reduction in R wave amplitude. Q waves are usually associated with myocardial necrosis but there is experimental evidence to suggest that myocardial damage may not be irreversible if there is early intervention (e.g. drugs, thrombolysis, angioplasty). Q waves are not specific for acute myocardial infarction, as they are also seen in left ventricular hypertrophy, cardiomyopathy, and rarely in association with myocardial tumours. In one third of patients the Q waves resolve within 18 months of acute infarction.

   Formerly, it was assumed that Q waves indicated transmural infarction. Patients who showed significant elevation in cardiac enzymes together with ST segment shift, but no Q waves were said to have sustained a subendocardial infarct. It is now clear that the relationship between the ECG evidence of full thickness or subendocardial infarction and the pathological findings is not absolute. A proportion of the 20% or so of patients who have a documented infarct without Q waves have an infarct in an area that is electrically silent to the 12 lead surface ECG.

Myocardial scintigraphy

Infarct avid myocardial scintigraphy is capable of accurately diagnosing and localising an acute myocardial infarct in the majority of patients. Furthermore, a semiquantitative assessment of the size of an infarct is possible, together with an estimation of the likely complication rate and mortality associated with a particular lesion. The short half-life of ^{99m}Tc-pyrophosphate makes it the radionuclide of choice; less than 5% remains in the blood after injection, 50% of the agent is extracted by bone and the remainder is excreted by the kidneys. Radionuclide is taken up by areas of myocardium where free calcium ions have accumulated within irreversibly damaged myocardial cells. The amount of uptake is proportional to the degree of myocardial damage, and is inversely related to the amount of flow reduction.

Imaging in multiple views can be undertaken in the coronary care unit using a portable scintillation camera 1–3 hours after intravenous injection of the radionuclide. A positive scan may be seen as early as 4 hours after the onset of symptoms and peaks at 48–72 hours. Extension of an infarct cannot be diagnosed with certainty because some patients do not have a positive scan until 6 days after the initial event. Focal areas of uptake are more specific than diffuse uptake and transmural infarcts can be more reliably detected than partial thickness infarction. Overall, the sensitivity is 90–95%, the specificity 80–85% and the predictive accuracy 85–90% for a transmural infarct. The specificity falls to 50% for subendocardial infarcts. ^{99m}Tc-pyrophospate imaging also has a role in the diagnosis of peroperative myocardial infarction complicating myocardial revascularisation procedures. Focal uptake of radionuclide (false positives) may also occur in left ventricular aneurysm, valvular calcification, myocardial contusion and following DC cardioversion.

Echocardiography

Both M-mode and cross-section echocardiography can be used in the assessment of acute myocardial infarction. The fast repetition rate and therefore superior images acquired with the M-mode technique are offset by the limited area of the myocardium that can be visualised at any one time. Large areas of the heart, for example the apex of the left ventricle, cannot be reliably seen using M-mode echocardiography. This limitation is particularly significant in ischaemic heart disease because the abnormalities of wall motion are localised (segmental), and not global. Cross-sectional echocardiography allows visualisation of all segments of the left ventricle and most of the right ventricle as well. Abnormal wall motion seen in any one view can be confirmed by imaging the same area in a different view and alterations in wall motion brought about by drug intervention can be followed by sequential studies.

Echocardiographic features of myocardial infarction

1. *Wall motion*

   Segmental abnormalities of wall motion demonstrable by echocardiography include hypokinesis, dyskinesis and akinesis. Incoordination of contraction and relaxation can be detected by recording a high quality M-mode echocardiogram with simultaneous apex- and phonocardiogram.

2. *Wall thickness*

   Lack of posterior wall and septal thickening during ventricular systole and a failure to thin during early diastole may indicate ischaemia. Scar tissue appears thin and functionally inert throughout the cardiac cycle.

3. *Cavity dimensions*

   Multiple myocardial infarcts can result in a dilated left ventricle with global impairment of systolic function which is indistinguishable from the ventricle of dilated cardiomyopathy.

4. *Echo texture*

   Myocardial fibrosis alters the acoustic properties of the myocardium. Areas of fibrosis and scarring appear as 'bright' areas of increased echodensity.

5. *Mural thrombus*

   Left ventricular thrombi can frequently be seen overlying areas of abnormal wall motion. They may be firmly attached to the underlying endocardium or alternatively they move back and forth when visualised in real time. Large thrombi appear alarming but there is no clear relationship between the presence of thrombi visualised by echocardiography and the likelihood of systemic embolism.

6. *Coronary artery imaging*

   Proximal coronary artery lesions, particularly those involving the left main stem have been visualised by echocardiography. The examination is technically difficult and time consuming and has no role in the evaluation of coronary artery disease in clinical practice.

7. *Complications of myocardial infarction*

   Acute mitral regurgitation, ventricular septal defect, myocardial rupture and left ventricular aneurysm can all be identified by echocardiography (see p. 39–41).

DIFFERENTIAL DIAGNOSIS

1. *Aortic dissection*
   Retrosternal pain radiating through to the back. Clinical evidence of absent or reduced pulses ± aortic regurgitation. Diagnosis confirmed with echocardiography, thoracic CT and cineangiography (see Ch. 10).

2. *Acute pericarditis*
   Chest pain relieved by sitting forward. Previous viral infection, systemic upset, friction rub and typical ECG (see Ch. 13).

3. *Acute pulmonary embolism*
   Marked breathlessness. Central chest pain inconspicuous, although pleuritic pain and haemoptysis may accompany peripheral emboli. Elevated venous pressure, right-sided third heart sound ± pleural rub. Arterial hypoxaemia. Pulmonary oligaemia on chest radiograph. Typical ECG. Embolism confirmed with V/Q scan or pulmonary arteriography (see Ch. 14).

4. *Chest wall pain*
   Superficial, localised pain, which may be precipitated by activity, and relieved by changes in position. Often fleeting lasting only a few seconds, and rarely central. Trigger points found on palpation. Particularly common after sternotomy. Improves with reassurance and minor analgesics.

5. *Tietze's syndrome*
   Uncommon. Painful swelling over the costochondral junctions. No systemic disturbance. Localised tenderness may be elicited, particularly over the second costochondral junction. Symptomatic treatment with minor analgesics and anti-inflammatory agents. Occasionally a local injection of corticosteroids may be necessary.

6. *Gastrointestinal disorders*
   Hiatus hernia and oesophageal reflux, oesophageal spasm or rupture, acute cholecystitis, peptic ulceration or acute pancreatitis may all cause diagnostic difficulty when considering acute myocardial infarction. A careful clinical history and appropriate tests (e.g. Barium meal, serum amylase, cholecystogram, upper gastrointestinal endoscopy) usually clarify the diagnosis. Oral nitrates may relieve the pain of oesophageal spasm. Some gastrointestinal conditions (e.g. pancreatitis, cholecystitis) may be associated with repolarisation abnormalities (ST/T changes) on the ECG.

TREATMENT OF UNCOMPLICATED MYOCARDIAL INFARCTION

1. *General measures*

   Once admitted to hospital the patient should be rapidly transferred to a coronary care unit (CCU). Time wasted in a casualty department, in X-ray, or undergoing a formal admitting procedure may result in life threatening arrhythmias occurring when the patient is not being monitored and has no vascular access. It is preferable for the patient with a diagnosis of possible infarction to be admitted to a CCU and then transferred to a general ward should the diagnosis prove to be incorrect. A system for the general practitioner to admit patients directly to the CCU is ideal.

   On admission to the CCU, the patient is attached to a (central) cardiac monitor. A large-bore needle (e.g. Venflon) is inserted into a vein for access and flushed with heparin. Central venous cannulation is not necessary as a routine procedure, but may be required (together with PA and systemic arterial monitoring) in some high risk patients (see p. 37). Blood is drawn for electrolytes, urea, creatinine, full blood count and cardiac enzymes. A portable (AP) chest radiograph is taken, together with a 12 lead ECG on a daily basis.

   A light diet is advisable because of possible nausea provoked by medication and the risk of inhalation following possible cardiac arrest. Similarly, a stool softener (e.g. Dorbanex, Dulcolax) should be given as a routine. In the absence of complications the patient may be transferred to a high dependency area of the general ward on the third day and discharged from hospital on the seventh day.

2. *Analgesia*

   Adequate analgesia is crucial in patients following acute myocardial infarction. Not only does uncontrolled pain cause the patient distress, but the associated increase in circulating catecholamines may provoke subendocardial ischaemia and arrhythmias. Opiates are the drugs of choice, either diamorphine (2.5–5.0 mg IV) or morphine sulphate (5–10 mg IV). Frequent small doses of intravenous opiates should be administered in order to keep the patient pain free because oral or intramuscular analgesics may be erratically absorbed. Opiate induced dilatation of the venous capacitance vessels, and to a lesser extent the systemic arterioles, may be particularly helpful in patients with pulmonary oedema.

   Side-effects are uncommon but include nausea and vomiting which should be treated prophylactically with prochlorperazine 10 mg, cyclizine 50 mg or metoclopramide 10 mg. Systemic hypotension is uncommon in patients treated in the supine position. Patients usually require opiates for 24–48 hours, but severe pain may recur with extension of the infarct or pericarditis.

2. *Bed rest*

   Limitation in physical activities is only necessary as long as the patient is in pain. Gradual mobilisation from 24–36 hours is the norm, with the patient sitting in a chair for short periods on the second day and taking short walks by the fourth day. Many patients find the use of a bedpan distressing, and a commode at the bedside is preferable. Isometric stress (e.g. lifting, stretching, bending) should be avoided.

3. *Sedation*

   Routine use of sedatives is unnecessary, but in patients who are particularly anxious, a short acting benzodiazepine (e.g. Lorazepam 1–2 mg three times daily and at night) may be helpful. Explanation and reassurance are important in helping to increase confidence.

4. *Oxygen*

   Little objective data support the routine use of supplemental oxygen following myocardial infarction. However, many patients experience psychological benefit from oxygen and for this reason it is widely prescribed. Nasal cannulae with 2–4 l/min humidified oxygen is convenient, although oxygen delivery is variable using this apparatus. In patients with evidence of pulmonary oedema, oxygen should be administered according to arterial blood gas estimations to maintain the $PaO_2 > 8kPa$. The usual precautions regarding the use of oxygen in patients with additional chronic airflow obstruction apply after acute myocardial infarction.

5. *Nitrates*

   Nitrates given by intravenous infusion (e.g. nitroglycerine, isosorbide dinitrate), sublingually (e.g. glyceryl trinitrate) or by cutaneous topical absorption (e.g. Transiderm-Nitro) may be effective in relieving ischaemic chest pain, particularly when used in combination with opiates.

   Beneficial haemodynamic consequences of nitrates include venous and arteriolar dilatation, coronary dilatation, and relief of coronary spasm. Nitrates also reduce LV volume and cardiac work, improve coordination of contraction and relaxation, and increase ventricular compliance. Routine use of intravenous nitrates as a means of improving left ventricular function following acute myocardial infarction are likely to become more generally used in the future. Experimental and clinical studies indicate that infarct size may be limited with intravenous nitrates (as measured by CPK.MB release, precordial ST segment mapping and ^{201}Tl scintigraphy), and the incidence of late arrhythmias and infarct extension is reduced. Side effects include headache, sinus tachycardia and systemic hypotension. A combination of nitrates and diuretics may be particularly potent in causing hypotension as a result of their combined effects in reducing preload.

6. *Beta blockade*

Beta blockers reduce heart rate, systemic blood pressure and cardiac output. Cardiac work and peak dp/dt are lowered, hence there is a reduction in myocardial oxygen consumption (MVO_2). The role of beta blockade very early after myocardial infarction is under debate and cannot be generally recommended at present. Evidence suggesting that beta blocking drugs favourably alter the prognosis following acute infarction indicates that treatment should be started early (<4 hours after the onset of chest pain), preferably by intravenous administration. Side effects appear surprisingly uncommon, even in patients with left severe ventricular dysfunction. Beta blockers should not be given to patients with high grade atrioventricular block, systemic hypotension, marked sinus bradycardia, or overt pulmonary oedema.

The benefits of using beta blocking drugs as a measure in secondary prevention are more compelling. A 25–30% reduction in late mortality can be expected due to a reduction in sudden death, arrhythmias and reinfarction. As with any Chronic treatment, the potential benefits have to be balanced against unwanted side-effects, particularly as the proportion of patients at risk probably constitutes no more than 10% of the total. Present data suggest that beta blockers should be commenced on day 4 or 5, and continued for 1–2 years. In the long-term, patients are more likely to adhere to a once daily drug regimen and fewer side-effects can be expected from a cardioselective preparation (e.g. Atenolol).

7. *Anticoagulants*

The underlying disturbance in the majority of patients sustaining a myocardial infarct is coronary thrombosis; this, coupled with the significant incidence of venous thrombosis and systemic embolism from mural thrombus, forms the theoretical basis for the use of anticoagulants. However, the use of anticoagulants in these circumstances is controversial. There is clear evidence that low dose subcutaneous heparin (5000 units three times daily) reduces the incidence of deep vein thrombosis and pulmonary embolism following myocardial infarction, but the indications for full anticoagulation with heparin or warfarin are less certain. Formal anticoagulation should probably be reserved for patients in cardiogenic shock, those who have sustained an arterial embolism to a major vessel, and patients in whom a large area of dyskinesis, left ventricular aneurysm or mural thrombus has been visualised by echocardiography or myocardial scintigraphy. In these patients, a continuous infusion of Heparin (40 000 units/24 h) is commenced, and the dose adjusted to maintain the KCT at 2–2.5x normal. When the patient is fully mobile, warfarin is added, and the heparin is discontinued once the dose of warfarin is therapeutic.

8. *Antiplatelet agents*

Few data support the routine use of antiplatelet agents (aspirin, dipyridamole, sulfinpyrazone) either in the early post-infarction period or as a secondary preventative measure. Side effects (particularly related to the gastrointestinal tract) may be intolerable, and the dose-dependent effects of aspirin on the thromboxane A2 (vasoconstrictor) and prostacyclin (vasodilator) pathways makes the interpretation and comparison of the available literature difficult.

9. *Other cardioactive drugs*

Up to 50% of patients admitted with an acute myocardial infarct are already taking cardioactive drugs for pre-existing angina or systemic hypertension. Beta blockers and calcium antagonists should be continued unless there is a specific indication for them to be stopped (e.g. systemic hypotension, bradycardia). It is advisable to discontinue diuretics as they may lead to electrolyte disturbance, and to reintroduce them if there is a specific indication for their use.

COMPLICATIONS

Arrhythmias

See Chapter 16.

Cardiogenic shock

'Shock' is a condition in which the cardiac output is inadequate to maintain vital organ function. The patient with cardiogenic shock as a consequence of myocardial infarction usually has less than 40% of viable myocardium, and the mortality in these circumstances exceeds 80%. Early recognition is important if intervention is to improve the otherwise dismal prognosis.

Features of cardiogenic shock

1. Systemic hypotension (systolic BP <90 mmHg). It should be noted that *perfusion* is more important than pressure, and perfusion may be adequate with a systolic BP <90 mmHg if the patient is on vasodilators
2. Low cardiac output (cardiac index <2.0 l/min/m²)
3. Impaired cerebral function: confusion, restlessness, drowsiness, secondary to poor cerebral perfusion
4. Oliguria (<20 ml urine/h)
5. Metabolic acidosis.

Using the above definition, less than 10% of patients who reach hospital are in cardiogenic shock as a complication of acute myocardial infarction. Treatment of cardiogenic shock aims at reducing myocardial oxygen demands without lowering cardiac output to such an extent that vital organ function is impaired.

Effective management of a patient in cardiogenic shock cannot be achieved outside an intensive care unit. Indwelling arterial, central venous, pulmonary arterial and urinary catheters are required in order to optimise fluid loading and pharmacological support.

Management

1. *Loading*
   If PACWP is low, infuse N. saline or plasma protein fraction (PPF) until it increases to 15–20 mmHg. Over enthusiastic diuresis may have lowered preload such that LV filling is inadequate. Patients with infarction involving both ventricles may require special treatment (see p. 44).
2. *Oxygenation*
   Maintain adequate (PaO₂<8 kPa) with supplemental oxygen, and assisted ventilation if necessary.
3. *Acid-base balance*
   Aim to correct severe metabolic acidosis (pH <7.3) with sodium bicarbonate if the PACWP is not too high. LV function improves if the pH is within the normal range, but the sodium load may precipitate pulmonary oedema.
4. *Anti-arrhythmic drugs*
   Premature contractions and episodes of sustained tachyarrhythmias reduce cardiac output. Appropriate anti-arrhythmic agents (see Ch. 16) should be administered having previously corrected acid-base and electrolyte disturbances in the knowledge that all these drugs may depress myocardial function to a variable degree.
5. *Diuretics*
   An elevated LV filling pressure (PACWP >25 mmHg) may be treated with diuretics which reduce pulmonary venous congestion and may improve oxygenation (see Ch. 5).

6. *Vasodilators*
   Arteriolar, venous and combination vasodilators are used to reduce 'preload', reduce systemic vascular resistance ('afterload') and increase tissue perfusion as appropriate (see Ch. 7).

7. *Inotropic agents*
   Inotropic drugs may need to be given in combination with vasodilators to maintain cardiac output, with the risk of provoking arrhythmias and increasing myocardial oxygen consumption.

8. *Intra-aortic balloon counterpulsation (IABC)*
   Approximately 10% of patients survive an episode of cardiogenic shock when treated with appropriate intravenous fluids, together with a combination of vasodilator and inotropic drugs. In centres equipped with IABC, mechanical assistance should be instituted when adequate doses of pharmacological agents have failed to improve the haemodynamic situation within 60 min. IABC improves left ventricular function by reducing afterload and cardiac work, hence reducing myocardial oxygen consumption. Counterpulsation also increases coronary perfusion and systemic output. An attempt should be made to wean the patient off the device within 24 hours. If mechanical assistance is required for more than 48 hours the prognosis is very poor, particularly in patients with no surgically remediable disease (e.g. VSD, acute mitral regurgitation, LV aneurysm).
   In a few centres, early myocardial revascularisation or resection of the infarct has been undertaken with reasonable success.

Acute mitral regurgitation

Partial papillary muscle rupture is an uncommon (<1%) complication of acute myocardial infarction. Papillary muscles are supplied by end-arteries and therefore vulnerable to ischaemic insult. Transection of a papillary muscle usually results in catastrophic mitral regurgitation and sudden death; therefore, partial rupture is seen more frequently in clinical practice. Postero-medial papillary muscle rupture in association with inferior infarction is more common than involvement of the antero-lateral papillary muscle. The appearance of a systolic thrill, loud pansystolic murmur and third heart sound heard widely over the precordium, together with the signs of acute pulmonary oedema during the first 10 days after infarction should alert the physician to the diagnosis. Post-infarction mitral regurgitation and ventricular septal defect cannot be differentiated on clinical grounds. Echocardiography shows the posterior mitral leaflet to be flail, prolapsing into the left atrium during systole. Cardiac catheterisation confirms an elevated PACWP, with a prominent 'v' wave, and severe mitral regurgitation is demonstrated by cineangiography. Without surgery 75% of patients are dead within 24 hours. Early surgical intervention (mitral valve replacement or repair) is associated with a reasonable prognosis if left ventricular function is not severely compromised.

Ventricular septal defect

Septal rupture accounts for 1–2% of deaths following myocardial infarction. It usually occurs as a consequence of anterior myocardial infarction involving the apical region of the septum, often in association with a left ventricular aneurysm. Physical signs are similar to those of acute mitral regurgitation (see p. 39). The diganosis can be confirmed at the bedside by detecting a step-up in oxygen saturation between right atrium and right ventricle using a Swan-Ganz flow directed catheter (see Ch. 20). Cross-sectional echocardiography frequently demonstrates the septal defect and cardiac catheterisation may be required to document the coronary artery anatomy prior to surgical intervention. Intravenous vasodilators (e.g. nitroprusside) and/or intra-aortic ballon counter-pulsation are best instituted prior to invasive investigation in view of the risks of cardiac catheterisation in this group. Surgery (repair of VSD ± aneurysmectomy ± coronary artery bypass grafting) should be undertaken early before the patient develops multisystem failure as a consequence of a low cardiac output. Operative mortality is 20–30% and right ventricular function appears to be an important determinant of long-term survival.

Cardiac rupture

10–15% of patients dying from myocardial infarction die from cardiac rupture. Rupture of the heart is more more common in the elderly, in females, and following extensive transmural infarction of the anterior free wall of the left ventricle. As death is usually sudden due to acute tamponade, there are few reports of successful intervention. Rarely, a small defect may be sealed off with organising thrombus and pericardium tissue, so called pseudoaneurysm.

Systemic embolism

Up to 50% of patients dying of acute myocardial infarction are found to have mural thrombus within the heart, most commonly in the apical region of the left ventricle. Thrombus is particularly common in patients with extensive transmural infarction or left ventricular aneurysm. Despite this, systemic embolism is seen in less than 5% of patients. Of these, at least 50% of emboli pass to the cerebral circulation, and the remainder involve the other major arteries including the renal, splenic, and mesenteric vessels. Emboli affecting the limbs may be amenable to removal by means of a balloon (Fogarty) catheter. Patients who develop emboli should be treated with a continuous infusion of heparin for 7 days, monitored according to the KCT and then switched to warfarin which is continued for 3 months. The efficacy of anticoagulants in these circumstances is uncertain. Recurrent thromboembolism is one of the indications for resection of a left ventricular aneurysm.

Post-myocardial infarction syndrome

Dressler's syndrome consisting of pleuro-pericarditis, fever, elevated ESR and leucocytosis occurs in 5–10% of patients following myocardial infarction. The condition has an immune basis, and although anti-myocardial antibodies can be detected, these are non-specific. Symptoms occur 2–6 weeks after infarction and the patients who develop this syndrome have not necessarily suffered from early pericarditis. The ECG has the typical appearance of acute pericarditis, the cardiac silhouette is enlarged on the chest radiograph, and echocardiography shows a small to moderate pericardial effusion. One third of patients have radiological evidence of bilateral pulmonary infiltrates. Aspirin or proprionic acid derivatives (NSAID), and occasionally a short course of corticosteroids will be required. The condition may recur, and rare cases of cardiac tamponade have been reported.

Left ventricular aneurysm

A ventricular aneurysm occurs as a late consequence of extensive transmural myocardial infarction and is characterised by a discrete area of thin and scarred myocardium that moves paradoxically. 80% are apical involving the territory of the left anterior descending coronary artery and the remainder are inferior. A history of recurrent chest pain, breathlessness, intractable arrhythmias or thromboembolism is typical. Clinical examination may reveal cardiac enlargement, a pre-systolic bulge medial to the apex beat and a third heart sound. Persistent ST segment elevation is present in most patients but this may merely indicate severe ischaemic ventricular disease rather than a discrete aneurysm. Similarly, the chest radiograph may reveal a discrete bulge (sometimes calcified) on the left heart border but this finding is unreliable. Cross-sectional echocardiography or gated blood pool scanning may show the aneurysm but the diagnosis can only be made with certainty using cineangiography. As many aneurysms are amenable to surgical resection, left ventricular cineangiography together with coronary arteriography should be undertaken in all patients suspected of having an aneurysm. An in-hospital mortality of 5% should be expected following aneurysm resection. Patients presenting with breathlessness fare less well with resection than the other subgroups.

REHABILITATION

The aim of rehabilitation is to integrate the patient back into society, and to encourage him to lead as normal life as possible. Rehabilitation programmes are tailored to individual requirements based on the age of the patient, their physical condition prior to infarction, and whether the infarct was well tolerated, or associated with complications.

Assuming the infarct was uncomplicated, a number of guidelines apply:

1. Explanation and reassurance both to the patient and their spouse are important in the development of realistic expectations.
2. Dietary advise is given, particularly concerning the avoidance of weight gain, and the importance of stopping smoking should be emphasized.
3. A progressive increase in physical activity is to be encouraged.
4. Emphasis should be on dynamic (isotonic) exercise (e.g. walking, swimming, cycling), rather than isometric exercise (e.g. lifting). Isometric stress causes a disproportionate increase in peripheral resistance and systemic blood pressure, whereas dynamic exercise leads to a gradual increase in heart rate and cardiac output, and encourages cardiac 'conditioning'.
5. If facilities are available, formal rehabilitation programmes and group activities should be encouraged as these allow patients to meet with others and discuss their similar problems.
6. A discussion on sexual activity is too often neglected, and this area may cause inappropriate concern to the patient.
7. Patients in all but the most strenuous jobs should return to work (part-time if necessary) within 8–12 weeks of the acute event. The longer the patient is away from work, the less likely they are to return. Driving for short distances can be commenced four weeks after an uncomplicated infarct.

PROGNOSIS

The overall mortality in acute myocardial infarction is approximately 40%, and half of these patients die within the first two hours of the onset of chest pain, frequently prior to reaching hospital. 30% of patients develop recurrent ischaemic chest pain whilst in hospital, and extension of the infarct occurs in 10–30%. Patients who are shown to have chest pain in association with ST/T changes in areas distant to the original lesion fare less well (by a factor of two), than patients who have repolarisation abnormalities in the area of the original infarct. Following discharge from hospital, 20% of patients die within the first year, and half of these are dead within 3 months.

Other determinants of a poor prognosis include:
1. Men >60 years old
2. Previous acute myocardial infarction
3. Previous history of angina, systemic hypertension, diabetes mellitus
4. Impaired LV function at the time of admission:
   Third heart sound, mitral regurgitation
   Radiographic cardiac enlargement ± pulmonary oedema
   Widespread changes on the ECG (Q wave and/or persistent ST/T changes)
   Peak CPK.MB >2000 IU
   Increased PACWP
   Reduced ejection fraction or increased end systolic volume on gated blood pool scanning
5. Arrhythmias:
   New atrial fibrillation.
   Frequent VPBs
   Complex VPBs (bigemini, multiform, salvos, R on T)
6. Heart block:
   Bifascicular, trifascicular
   2° AV block (Mobitz II)
   3° (complete) AV block.

EXERCISE TESTING FOLLOWING ACUTE MYOCARDIAL INFARCTION

Early treadmill exercise testing and 24 hour ECG tape monitoring has recently been introduced in an attempt to identify high risk subgroups.

A pre-discharge (or six week) symptom limited treadmill exercise test should be a routine procedure in survivors of acute myocardial infarction providing:
1. Patient is mobile and without chest pain
2. No evidence of impaired myocardial function at rest (e.g. tachycardia, pulmonary oedema etc.)
3. No ventricular arrhythmias.

A poor prognosis in terms of survival and the incidence of further 'events' (e.g. sudden death, recurrent angina, further infarction etc.) can be predicted if one or more of the following occur on exercise:
1. Chest pain (angina pectoris)
2. Poor haemodynamic response
3. ST segment depression

        4. Exercise-induced ventricular arrhythmias
        5. Exercise-induced ST segment elevation.
Patients in these high-risk subgroups should undergo coronary
arteriography six weeks after the acute event (see Ch. 3).

RIGHT VENTRICULAR INFARCTION

Clinical recognition of right ventricular infarction is difficult, and
frequently missed because it is not considered as a clinical entity. This
situation may be compounded by the misinterpretation of physical signs
which results in inappropriate management. Infarction of the right
ventricle should be considered in any patient who has ECG evidence of
inferior infarction (ST segment elevation and/or Q waves in leads II, III
and aVF).

    Right ventricular infarction usually involving the posterior wall always
occurs as a result of a lesion in the right coronary artery. Isolated
infarction of the right ventricle is uncommon, accounting for less than
5% of infarcts found at autopsy, although it may be seen in association
with 30–50% of infarcts affecting the left ventricle particularly those
involving the inferior wall. The extent of right ventricular damage is
determined by the pattern of coronary blood supply. In 85% of patients
the posterior descending coronary artery is a branch of the right coronary
artery and it is this group of patients who are at highest risk from an
isolated infarct of the right ventricle. In the remaining patients there is
an additional blood supply from the left circumflex to the posteroinferior
region of the right ventricle. Dual blood supply to the anterior wall of
the right ventricle (RCA and branches of the LAD) make infarction of
this region very rare.

Physical signs

        1. *Elevated venous pressure*
           Prominent 'a' wave, steep 'x' and 'y' descents, with dominant
           'y'. Inability of the right ventricle to increase stroke volume
           in response to the increase in venous return during
           inspiration causes an inappropriate increase in the venous
           pressure during inspiration — Kussmaul's sign.
        2. *Right sided S4 and S3*
        3. *Absence of pulmonary oedema*
        4. *Systemic hypotension*

Investigations

ECG features of an inferior infarct are seen in most patients and the
addition of a right precordial lead (V$_4$R) may be useful in patients

thought to have right ventricular infarction. Bedside monitoring (see Ch. 20) and myocardial scintigraphy (^{99m}Tc pyrophosphate) are the only methods of diagnosing right ventricular infarction with certainty, or assessing the contribution of right ventricular infarction in patients who have an infarct involving both ventricles. Haemodynamics of right ventricular infarction:

1. Elevated RA pressure
2. Elevated RVEDP ± low RV systolic pressure
3. Low/normal PA pressure
4. Low/normal PACWP
5. Low cardiac output

Differential diagnosis

1. *Pericardial tamponade*
   No chest pain. Elevated venous pressure with dominant 'x' descent. Arterial paradox. Equal RA pressure and PACWP. Normal cardiac enzymes. Effusion confirmed by echocardiography (see Ch. 13).
2. *Pericardial constriction*
   No chest pain. Elevated venous pressure, visible 'x' and 'y' descents, 'y' dominant (usually). Similar pressures in all four cardiac chambers (RA, RVEDP, PACWP, LVEDP). Normal cardiac enzymes (see Ch. 13).
3. *Restrictive cardiomyopathy*
   No chest pain. Physical sign and haemodynamics similar to pericardial constriction. Confirm diagnosis with endomyocardial biopsy and echocardiography (see Ch. 6).
4. *Massive pulmonary embolism*
   Elevated venous pressure. Breathlessness, pain may be absent. Arterial hypoxaemia. Confirm with V/Q scan or pulmonary arteriography (see Ch. 14)

Management

Patients who have sustained an infarct of the right ventricle require a high venous filling pressure ('preload'). The tendency to treat the patient with diuretics because the venous pressure is elevated is inappropriate. Ideal fluid management can only be achieved using PA monitoring.

Crystalloid (e.g. N.Saline) or plasma protein fraction (PPF) should be infused to maintain an adequate cardiac output which can be confirmed with a flow-directed (Swan-Ganz) thermodilution catheter. A PACWP as high as 15–20 mmHg may be required but great care is needed to avoid precipitating pulmonary oedema particularly as most patients have additional left ventricular dysfunction.

When LV 'preload' is adequate inotropic support and/or vasodilators may be required if the cardiac output remains low. Agents that lower 'preload' by their action on venous capacitance vessels should be avoided if possible (e.g. nitrates, nitroprusside), and opiates (which also have a venodilator action) must be used with care. An infusion of salbutamol, phentolamine or hydrallazine is appropriate, and if inotropic support is needed then dobutamine is preferred over dopamine because of the lack of alpha agonist action. Pulmonary vascular resistance can be minimised by the administration of oxygen.

Complications of right ventricular infarction include mural thrombus and pulmonary embolism, septal rupture, and tricuspid regurgitation secondary to a dilated annulus or papillary muscle ischaemia.

There are too few studies to estimate the prognosis of patients with right ventricular infarction although it is clear that the acute mortality of an inferior infarct is approximately half that of an anterior infarct.

PRE-HOSPITAL MANAGEMENT OF ACUTE MYOCARDIAL INFARCTION

In the United Kingdom, 50% of patients die from acute myocardial infarction without seeing a doctor. Thus, studies comparing home and hospital management of acute myocardial infarction are actually comparing the results of selected populations of survivors. Survival statistics are very much dependent on the efficiency of pre-hospital care, which in the UK is generally of a low standard except in certain areas (e.g. Belfast, Brighton). Within the first 30 minutes of the onset of chest pain 80% of patients experience a disturbance of cardiac rhythm. Bradyarrhythmias are particularly common in patients sustaining an inferior infarct and tachyarrhythmias occur predominantly in patients with anterior infarction. Not surprisingly, trials observing the efficacy of bystander-initiated cardiopulmonary resuscitation (CPR) and mobile coronary care ambulances manned by trained personnel (paramedics), have found them to be effective in reducing the early mortality associated with acute myocardial infarction.

Considerable progress has been made in some communities (e.g. Seattle), in which the majority of the public have undergone formal training, and are competent in the technique of CPR. In the future, emphasis is likely to be on the pre-hospital management of acute myocardial infarction, rather than increasing the numbers of coronary care facilities.

3. INTERVENTION IN PATIENTS WITH CORONARY ARTERY DISEASE

CORONARY ARTERIOGRAPHY

In experienced hands coronary arteriography is a safe technique with a morbidity of 2–3% and a mortality of <0.1% (see Ch. 20). Furthermore, it is currently the only method of accurately delineating coronary artery anatomy, and is therefore a necessary prerequisite to coronary artery bypass grafting, percutaneous coronary angioplasty and intracoronary thrombolysis.

In 1980, 100 coronary arteriograms were carried out per 100 000 of the population in the USA, and although the frequency of investigation is lower in the United Kingdom, the costs are still considerable. With the limited facilities available careful thought must be given to the indications for coronary arteriography. Indications for invasive investigation will differ from one centre to another, but there is a general consensus that coronary arteriography is appropriate in some groups of patients.

Indications for coronary arteriography

1. Intractable symptoms of coronary artery disease despite maximal medical treatment.

   This tends to be the major indication for coronary arteriography in the UK and in other countries where resources are limited. Persisting with medical treatment may be inappropriate in some patients because of time lost from work, side effects from medication, progressive left ventricular disease, and the improved survival when some subgroups of patients are treated surgically.

2. Determination of prognosis in a patient with known coronary artery disease.

   It has become clear that certain subgroups of patients have improved survival when treated surgically (see p. 60) and the severity of coronary artery disease can only be determined by arteriography.

3. Stable chest pain with marked ischaemic changes on exercise testing or a thallium study.

Patients with left ventricular dysfunction (dyskinesis, akinesis, or LV aneurysm) determined non-invasively by a thallium study, or who show an abnormal haemodynamic response or marked ST/T changes on exercise testing have a less favourable prognosis and warrant coronary arteriography.

4. Patients with chest pain in whom the aetiology is unclear.

A coronary arteriogram showing no organic disease may be particularly helpful and reassuring in the patient who is repeatedly admitted to hospital with episodes of recurrent chest pain.

5. Unstable angina.

Angina at rest (without enzyme evidence of myocardial infarction) that persists despite medical treatment is associated with a worse prognosis than stable angina and is therefore an indication for urgent arteriography. Definitive treatment may involve angioplasty, thrombolysis or early bypass grafting.

6. Post myocardial infarction.

Survivors of myocardial infarction can be stratified for risk according to the results of early exercise stress testing (see Ch. 2). Those in the high risk group should be investigated approximately 6 weeks after acute infarction. Other patients who should undergo coronary arteriography include young patients (>40 years) and any patient who develops recurrent chest pain following myocardial infarction.

7. Acute myocardial infarction.

In a few centres urgent intervention following myocardial infarction (i.e. <4 hours from the onset of chest pain) is feasible. Success has been reported using coronary angioplasty, thrombolysis, dissolution of coronary thrombus with a guide wire and coronary artery bypass grafting in these patients.

8. Survivors of near miss sudden death.

In 10% of patients the first manifestation of coronary artery disease is sudden death as a result of a ventricular arrhythmia. Coronary arteriography should be combined with electrophysiological testing in this group.

9. Symptoms following coronary artery bypass grafting.

With increasing numbers of patients undergoing coronary artery bypass grafting, recurrent chest pain following surgery is being seen more frequently. Pain within the first year after operation is usually related to incomplete revascularisation, graft occlusion or stenosis. As a result of increasing surgical expertise graft occlusion is usually related to poor distal runoff, rather than a technically inadequate anastomosis. Late recurrence of symptoms is either due to

progression of the coronary artery disease in the native
circulation or graft atherosclerosis.
10. Follow-up after coronary angioplasty or thrombolysis.
    Up to 30% of patients undergoing angioplasty or
    thrombolysis develop recurrent symptoms; at present follow-
    up arteriography at six months should be a routine
    procedure both as an internal audit and to determine the
    efficacy of the procedure.

In the West, coronary artery disease, which is frequently asymptomatic,
is present in 5% of middle aged men. In one study, 30% of
asymptomatic patients who were investigated by coronary arteriography
developed symptoms within 8 years. The initial manifestation of coronary
artery disease is sudden death in 10% of patients and acute myocardial
infarction in 40%. A case could be made therefore to screen middle-aged
men for coronary artery disease. In some areas of the USA this may be
happening, but in view of the expense involved it is unlikely that this
situation will arise in the UK and elsewhere. It would appear to be more
cost effective to channel resources into health education and primary
prevention. In certain subgroups however (e.g. airline pilots) the
indications for coronary arteriography will be more liberal than in the
general population.

Thrombolytic therapy

Thrombosis of a major coronary artery can usually be identified during
the first few hours of the evolution of an acute transmural myocardial
infarct. As a consequence of the sudden reduction in myocardial oxygen
supply, progressive myocardial necrosis occurs from about 15 minutes
and is complete within six hours. Experimental studies have shown that
the infusion of a thrombolytic agent can lyse the clot and that early
reperfusion is associated with a reduction in infarct size and improved
LV function.

Since 1957, numerous studies using intravenous agents have evaluated
the therapeutic usefulness of this approach. Early results were
inconsistent and in general the incidence of side effects was unacceptable.
Recently, the appreciation that coronary arteriography can be undertaken
at low risk whilst myocardial infarction is evolving has stimulated
enthusiasm for intracoronary thrombolysis.

Patient selection

Patients with evolving transmural infarction in whom thrombolysis can be
commenced within three hours of the onset of chest pain are ideal
candidates for this form of treatment. Typical chest pain with ST
segment elevation and reciprocal depression is very strongly correlated
with coronary thrombosis and transmural infarction. It has become clear

that the longer the patient has been symptomatic, the lower is the chance that a satisfactory result will be achieved. Unstable angina or subendocardial infarction does not respond favourably to thrombolysis.

Contraindications to thrombolysis include old age (>70 years), recent major surgery, recent cerebrovascular events, active gastrointestinal bleeding, bleeding diathesis and anaemia. Cardiogenic shock is not a contraindication to thrombolysis.

Thrombolytic agents

Streptokinase and urokinase are the two currently available thrombolytic agents approved for clinical use. Their mode of action is different. Streptokinase is a protein by-product of group C beta-haemolytic streptococci and activates the fibrinolytic system by combining with plasminogen to form an activator complex, which then converts plasminogen to plasmin. Plasmin is a proteolytic enzyme that lyses fibrin. Urokinase is non-antigenic and has a direct action on thrombolysis. The dose-effect relationship of urokinase is more predictable than streptokinase but it is also more costly. Most experience in the literature refers to streptokinase.

Local intracoronary infusion of streptokinase probably activates plasminogen bound to the thrombus and does not require systemic fibrinolysis, whereas intravenous thrombolysis requires the systemic degradation of fibrin with the production of fibrin split products (FDPs).

The recent development of lytic agents with the property of 'clot selectivity', for example, tissue-type plasminogen activator (t-PA) and acylated streptokinase-plasminogen complex, offer the promise of coronary thrombolysis from a peripheral vein injection without the unwanted consequences of systemic thrombolysis.

Intracoronary or intravenous?

The proponents of intracoronary administration point out that a lower total dose of streptokinase is required when compared with the intravenous route, the local concentration of the agent within the coronary artery is higher, and bleeding complications are seen less frequently. In any case coronary arteriography will be required to document the coronary anatomy and to confirm the result, therefore the streptokinase may as well be infused directly onto the lesion. Furthermore, if guide wire recanalisation, coronary angioplasty or intracoronary nitroglycerin is required after thrombolytic therapy, this can be undertaken with little additional effort (see p. 53).

Against this must be balanced the small but significant risk of undertaking coronary arteriography during evolving myocardial infarction, and more importantly, the delay in initiating thrombolysis because of the practical difficulties involved in arranging emergency cardiac catheterisation. Recent experience has shown that thrombolysis using the intravenous route may be associated with similar success rate to intracoronary thrombolysis without an increased incidence of side-effects. The analysis of serial ST segment changes may be used to monitor progress as a non-invasive alternative to coronary arteriography. If further studies confirm that the intravenous route is an acceptable alternative to the intracoronary approach the potential application of thrombolysis in acute myocardial infarction will be enormous.

Technique

1. *Intracoronary*

   Either the brachial or femoral approach maybe used, but the femoral route is preferred. A routine coronary arteriogram is undertaken using 8F Judkins catheters (see Ch. 20), following prior intravenous administration of heparin 10 000 IU, and hydrocortisone 200 mg. Streptokinase can either be infused into the coronary ostium through the regular coronary catheter, or selectively into the affected artery (in close proximity to the thrombus) via a 2F or 3F catheter passed through a high-flow Judkins catheter with an untapered tip.

   Intracoronary nitroglycerin (200 μm) is administered to reverse coronary spasm. This has little effect in the majority of patients with evolving myocardial infarction. An initial bolus of 10 000–20 000 IU of streptokinase is given, followed by a continuous infusion of 2000–6000 IU per minute. Limited coronary arteriography is repeated every 15 minutes to assess the state of the thrombus. Following dissolution of the clot, the infusion is reduced to 2000 IU per minute and continued for a further 30–60 minutes up to a maximum dose of 350 000 IU.

   After completion of the procedure the catheter is removed but the arterial and venous sheaths are left in situ in the groin. This allows immediate access should further intervention prove necessary, or insertion of a temporary pacing catheter be required. A coagulation profile is checked for evidence of systemic thrombolysis (thrombin time, reptilase time and FDPs). Full anticoagulation is then commenced wth an intravenous infusion of heparin to maintain the KCT at twice the control value (approximately 40 000 IU heparin per 24 hours), for 7–10 days, followed by warfarin for 3–6 months.

2. *Intravenous*

   An intravenous infusion of 500 000–1 500 000 IU over a 60 minute period is required to achieve thrombolysis in most patients. Success can be assessed non-invasively by monitoring the abrupt relief of chest pain, resolution of ST segment deviation, occurrence of specific reperfusion

arrhythmias, and confirmed with a follow-up coronary
arteriogram after three days. A loading dose of heparin
followed by an intravenous infusion (as above) should be
started as soon as the streptokinase has been discontinued.

Results

Successful reperfusion can be achieved in 75–85% of cases within 35
minutes. Lesions in the left circumflex artery appear to take significantly
longer to lyse than lesions in the left anterior descending or the right
coronary artery.

The beneficial effects of thrombolysis have been measured in terms of
a reduction in mortality, relief of chest pain, normalisation of ST
segment shift, and improvement in LV function. A 50% reduction in the
early hospital mortality from acute myocardial infarction (i.e. 10–20%
reduced to 5–10%) can be expected following thrombolysis. However, as
reocclusion rates are high (20–35%), salvage of ischaemic myocardium
during treatment of evolving myocardial infarction can only be regarded
as an interim measure.

Complications

1. *Bleeding*
   Major haemorrhage occurs in 1–2% of patients, and minor
   bleeding in up to 10%. Haemorrhage appears to be more
   common in patients who have had >200 000 IU of
   streptokinase, or when the fibrinogen level falls to
   <100 mg/dl. Leaving arterial and venous cannulae in situ
   significantly reduces the incidence of minor bleeding.
2. *Reperfusion arrhythmias*
   Up to 20% of patients experience reperfusion arrhythmias.
   Idioventricular rhythm and ventricular tachycardia are most
   commonly seen, but ventricular fibrillation has been reported
   in 10% of cases. Antiarrhythmic drugs are often ineffective,
   and sustained arrhythmias sufficient to cause haemodynamic
   compromise respond to DC countershock. Slow
   idioventricular rhythm or sinus bradycardia (complicating
   inferior or right ventricular infarction) may require temporary
   transvenous ventricular pacing.
3. *Reinfarction*
   Reinfarction occurs in 15–25% of patients, and is particularly
   common within the first four days after thrombolysis.
   Reinfarction usually results from thrombotic reocclusion, and
   repeat thrombolysis is effective in more than half the
   patients. The reinfarction rate may be reduced by early
   myocardial revascularisation (see p. 53).

4. *Myocardial haemorrhage*
This has been observed in patients dying early after thrombolysis, but its significance is unclear.

5. *Allergy to streptokinase*
Reactions to streptokinase are rare in patients pretreated with intravenous hydrocortisone 200 mg.

THROMBOLYSIS AND CORONARY ANGIOPLASTY

Coronary thrombosis frequently occurs in association with coronary atherosclerosis. A logical development in the field of coronary intervention is to combine intracoronary thrombolysis with percutaneous coronary angioplasty. At present it is not possible to assess the role of this technique on the preliminary data available.

THROMBOLYSIS AND CORONARY ARTERY BYPASS GRAFTING

Reocclusion is common after thrombolysis, and a number of studies have shown that early coronary artery bypass grafting can reduce the rate of reinfarction and improve LV function following the revascularisation of ischaemic myocardium.

Very early bypass grafting (i.e. on the day of thrombolysis) may be associated with bleeding complications but these are surprisingly rare. It is suggested that all intravenous and intraarterial cannulae are left in situ until after completion of the surgery and until such time as coagulation studies show no evidence of thrombolysis. Large quantities of fresh frozen plasma or cryoprecipitate may be required and are best administered in conjunction with a haematologist. Surgery performed three or more days after thrombolysis is not associated with increased risks.

PERCUTANEOUS CORONARY ANGIOPLASTY (PTCA)

Following the initial report of successful percutaneous dilatation of peripheral vascular lesions by Dotter in 1964, the technique was first applied to coronary arteries by Gruentzig in 1977. This application of the technique is therefore new, the indications and equipment are still evolving, and the follow-up necessarily short. There is however no doubt that PTCA is a considerable advance in selected patients. Whereas coronary angioplasty was first advocated for single, proximal, discrete, non-calcified lesions, recent reports have demonstrated that angioplasty may be effective in multiple, distal, calcified and segmental lesions, together with lesions in coronary bypass grafts.

Pathology

Animal and human studies indicate that the increase in the diameter of the coronary artery lumen following angioplasty is brought about by a number of mechanisms. In non-calcified lesions, dilatation occurs as a result of splitting of the intima and media. Fractures and tears in the atheromatous plaque can be seen and compression and compaction of the intima and extrusion of fluid may also be important factors. In eccentric calcified lesions the increase in lumen appears to be due to dilatation of the normal segment of the arterial wall with little change in the areas of calcification. Angioplasty may result in loss of endothelium but re-endothelialisation of the denuded area occurs within a few days.

In patients who develop recurrent lesions, intimal proliferation indistinguishable from de novo coronary atherosclerosis has been documented.

Indications

With increasing experience, the indications for PTCA are changing. In general, the criteria for accepting a candidate for PTCA are similar to CABG, that is, for relief of symptoms. In view of the possibility of the patient requiring urgent CABG as a consequence of PTCA, there is no place for the 'prophylactic' dilatation of minor lesions if they are not severe enough to warrant CABG. Furthermore, dilatation of minor lesions may be associated with recurrence, and the recurrence may be more severe than the original lesion.

1. *Single vessel disease*
   Single, proximal discrete lesions remain the ideal indication for PTCA, but these only account for 1–10% of all cases of coronary artery disease. Relief of symptoms is the primary indication, but some would favour dilating a high grade proximal left anterior descending lesion in a patient with an unfavourable exercise test or thallium study.

2. *Multiple lesions*
   The criteria for dilating multiple lesions (either sequential or in more than one vessel) remain to be defined. Dilatation of numerous lesions in a single patient is technically feasible, although there is some data to suggest that the primary success rate and complication rate may be higher in these patients.

3. *Coronary artery bypass grafts*
   PTCA has been successfully used to dilate lesions in the proximal, distal and body of coronary artery bypass grafts,

and with experience lesions within internal mammary grafts can also be dilated. Furthermore, graft runoff may be improved by dilating lesions in the distal native vessel. Although an acceptable primary success rate (up to 90%) is possible, the recurrence rate appears to be higher when compared with native lesions.

4. *Recurrent lesions*

   Approximately 30% of patients develop recurrent symptoms following PTCA, which usually correlate with recurrence of the stenosis. Many of these patients respond favourably to a second angioplasty.

5. *Other lesions*

   Preliminary results indicate that PTCA *may* be used in left main-stem disease, coronary artery occlusion, and in recent or evolving myocardial infarction (often in combination with thrombolysis).

Procedure

The principles involved in PTCA are simple, but considerable expertise is necessary in order to achieve a high degree of success with an acceptably low complication rate. Prior to commencing angioplasty a number of preliminaries should be carried out:

1. *Previous coronary arteriography*

   The patients must have undergone recent coronary arteriography and the lesion(s) appear suitable for PTCA.

2. *Exercise tolerance*

   An objective assessment of exercise capacity (e.g. treadmill test, or exercise thallium) prior to angioplasty serves as a useful baseline for comparison with post-angioplasty studies.

3. *Involvement of the cardiovascular surgeon*

   The coronary arteriograms should be reviewed by the cardiologist in consultation with the cardiac surgeon *prior* to commencing PTCA. Ideally, the surgeon should see the patient prior to angioplasty to confirm that he or she is a suitable candidate for CABG.

4. *Operating theatre standby*

   A full cardiac surgical team (cardiac surgeon and assistant, anaesthetist, perfusionist, scrub nurses etc.), should be standing by such that the patient can be placed on cardiopulmonary bypass within 15–30 minutes if necessary. Time is saved if the chest is shaved and prepared prior to commencing angioplasty, and the patient has blood cross-matched as for CABG.

5. *Consent*

   A detailed explanation of the risks and possible complications of the procedure, together with written informed consent for

PTCA and if necessary CABG. The catheterisation laboratory must be equipped with a high resolution image intensifier, together with the ability to simultaneously display high quality video freeze frames. A biplane facility is advantageous.

Technique

1. *Coronary arteriography*
   Routine coronary arteriography (see Ch. 20) is undertaken immediately prior to PTCA to ensure that the severity of the lesion(s) is unchanged. The right femoral approach using a 9F valved sheath is preferred. The lesion to be dilated is identified and visualised in several planes. Important side branches that may be occluded during balloon inflation are noted as is the anatomy of the distal vessels. Representative freeze frames are displayed on the monitor throughout the procedure for comparison. In the patient undergoing dilatation of the right coronary artery, or left circumflex artery with a left dominant system, the insertion of a 6F temporary pacing electrode in the right ventricle via the right femoral vein is a sensible precaution.

2. *Guiding catheter*
   An 8 or 9F guiding catheter is introduced through the valved sheath retrogradely into the ascending aorta. 10 000 units of heparin are administered intravenously, together with calcium antagonists and intravenous nitrates to minimise coronary spasm. The catheter is then advanced into position in the left or right coronary ostium such that coronary blood flow is not impaired.

3. *Balloon catheter*
   The appropriate balloon is selected and tested. Recent advances in balloon technology include a low-profile (1.04 mm diameter deflated, 2.00 mm inflated) balloon that is capable of withstanding pressures of 12–13 atmospheres. The double lumen balloon catheter is advanced through the guiding catheter to lie at the coronary artery ostium. Baseline pressures are recorded via the distal port.

4. *Guide wire*
   A high-torque monofilament guide wire 0.018 inches in diameter with a spring guided tip is passed through the balloon catheter and advanced down the coronary artery. As the lesion is approached, nitroglycerin (200 μg) is infused into the coronary artery to reduce spasm. Great care is taken in passing the guide wire over the lesion, particularly if resistance is encountered, as this may indicate that the tip of

the wire is under a plaque with the risk of possible dissection.

Once the tip of the wire is distal to the lesion it is left in situ. This has the effect of anchoring the system, and allows one or more balloons to be exchanged over the guide wire without further risk of dissection.

5. *Dilatation*

The balloon is advanced over the guide wire to bridge the lesion. The extremities of the balloon are indicated by gold markers which allow accurate positioning of the balloon in relation to the stenosis. Pressure in the distal coronary artery is measured through the distal port of the balloon. Simultaneous display of the pressure in the coronary ostium (via the guiding catheter) permits assessment of the gradient across the lesion.

Balloon distention is maintained for 10–60 s depending on the appearance of the lesion and the improvement in the gradient, and how well the inflation is tolerated by the patient (chest pain, systemic hypotension etc.). Symptoms during balloon dilatation may be controlled by nitrates infused into the coronary artery or intravenous opiates. Occasionally continuing angina responds to injection of (oxygen rich) arterial blood (obtained from the side-arm of the femoral artery sheath) into the distal coronary artery.

6. *Check arteriogram*

After dilatation is complete, coronary arteriograms are repeated with the guide wire left in situ, and finally with the guide wire removed to accurately assess the result. On no account should the guide wire be reintroduced once it has been removed.

7. *Completing the procedure*

Heparin is not reversed and should be continued for 24 hours. Both the arterial and venous sheaths are left in situ for 6 hours after the heparin is discontinued. This permits ready access to the arterial system should chest pain recur in the early post angioplasty period in which case coronary arteriography can be repeated. Early recurrence of chest pain is not infrequent and usually relates to coronary 'bruising' by the guide wire or balloon rather than dissection or coronary thrombosis. Serial ECG's and estimations of CPK.MB over the subsequent 48 hours will confirm or exclude myocardial infarction.

Primary success

The frequency of successful dilatation, defined as a reduction in the diameter of the stenosis by >20%, increases with experience. In centres that have performed <50 cases the primary success rate is approximately 60%, but this increases to 90% in the best centres. Primary success is highest in single vessel disease, particularly in lesions involving the left anterior descending artery, and non-calcified lesions are more successfully dilated than calcified lesions.

Complications

The incidence of complications relates to the degree of expertise and the 'learning curve' of the operator. Recent advances in catheter and guide wire design undoubtedly make for a safer procedure. Predictors of major complications include multivessel disease, eccentric and/or calcified lesions, long (>20 mm) stenoses and female gender.

1. *Death*
   The most important factors in preventing early death are the experience of the operator, together with the ability to perform efficient emergency bypass surgery. Early death rates vary from 0.07–3.2%.

   Patients at increased risk include the elderly, those with left main stem or multivessel disease, previous CABG or myocardial dysfunction. Patients who have previously sustained an acute myocardial infarction who are undergoing PTCA to another vessel which supplies blood to the bulk of the viable myocardium are a particularly high risk group. Late deaths are uncommon.

2. *Emergency coronary artery bypass surgery*
   Emergency CABG is indicated for coronary dissection or occlusion, coronary embolism, prolonged spasm or intractable chest pain. Experienced operators are becoming more willing to 'sit out' episodes of coronary artery occlusion secondary to spasm by administering large quantities of intracoronary nitrates. Similarly, coronary occlusion secondary to dissection may be amenable to redilatation to 'tack up' the flap if the guide wire has been left in situ. Overall, the incidence of emergency CABG is 2–7% in reported series.

3. *Acute myocardial infarction*
   The incidence of myocardial infarction varies from 0.5–5%, and the rate falls with experience and prompt revascularisation. Patients with long eccentric lesions closely related to major branches are particularly liable to acute infarction.

Drug therapy after angioplasty

Most centres advocate aspirin 75–300 mg daily to be taken as an antiplatelet agent after PTCA. A combination of aspirin and dipyridamole (100 mg four times daily) may be superior to aspirin alone and Nifedipine may also have a role in the early follow-up period.

Late follow-up and recurrence

Most patients with recurrent symptoms have recurrence of the stenosis. The overall incidence of recurrence is 30% over a six year follow-up period. Recurrent lesions are most common within the first six months, and therefore repeat coronary arteriography is advisable to document the coronary artery anatomy at that time. Silent restenosis is rare, and the results of stress testing after PTCA correlate closely with arteriographic evidence of recurrence.

Recurrence is more common with lesions of the left anterior descending, and in patients who have undergone multiple dilatations. Overall, 10–15% of patients will require repeat PTCA (or CABG) within the first 12 months for recurrent symptoms. The appearance of the lesion following dilatation (i.e. the 'quality' of the dilatation) is also an important factor, and the rate of recurrence is significantly lower in patients in whom a large diameter (3.5 mm) balloon was used together with a high (>8–9 atmospheres) inflation pressure.

Following single vessel PTCA, 5 year survival is 97%, and 88% at 4 years after multivessel PTCA. Predictors of late death include acute myocardial infarction prior to PTCA, left main stem stenosis, multivessel disease and male gender.

CORONARY ARTERY BYPASS GRAFTING

Attempts at cardiac denervation were first reported between 1910 and 1920, and although direct surgery on the coronary arteries was first performed by Bailey in 1957, it required the development of cardiopulmonary bypass and coronary arteriography before coronary artery bypass surgery became a routine procedure. Since the first successful report in 1976 there has been an explosion in coronary artery bypass grafting. Indeed, it has been estimated that the coronary artery bypass 'industry' in the USA costs approximately $3.3 billion per annum. By 1985, approximately 2 million coronary artery bypass operations had been carried out worldwide.

Over a similar period there have been major developments in the medical treatment of coronary artery disease (e.g. beta blockade, calcium antagonists, long-acting nitrates), together with the more recent use of PTCA and thrombolysis.

Only recently have the results of large prospective trials clearly documented the effects of surgical or medical therapy on the natural history of coronary artery disease, such that a rational decision can be made with regard to the optimal treatment for a particular patient.

Surgical vs medical treatment

1. *Single vessel disease*

   Lesions of the proximal left anterior descending coronary artery (that is, prior to the first septal perforator) have a worse prognosis than more distal lesions. Single vessel disease involving the distal LAD, left circumflex and right coronary artery have a similar five year survival of 91–96% whether treated medically or surgically. The attrition rate for single vessel disease is approximately 2% per annum. LV function is a major determinant of survival and in patients with an ejection fraction of <50% the five year survival falls to 81–83%. Furthermore, relief of angina is not significantly different in those patients treated medically or surgically.

   In isolated lesions of the proximal LAD, the five year mortality is 10%, which is considerably higher than the mortality for isolated distal LAD lesions. This difference probably relates to the amount of myocardium in jeopardy should sudden occlusion take place.

   Operative mortality in patients with single vessel disease (including patients with proximal LAD lesions) should approach 0%.

2. *Two vessel disease*

   Survival with two vessel disease is similar in patients treated medically and surgically, with 88–96% alive at five years. However, patients with a proximal LAD lesion in association with disease of one other vessel are better treated with surgery (five year survival 93% with surgery, compared to 82% with medical treatment).

   Not only does LV function affect long-term survival, but patients with impaired LV function (ejection fraction <50%) have a higher operative mortality than those with normal function (3.3% vs 0.5%).

3. *Triple vessel disease*

   CABG is the procedure of choice in this group, with a five year survival of 94%, falling to 90% if LV function is impaired. Survival is similar if patients with triple vessel disease and normal LV function are treated medically, but up to 40% cross over to the surgical group over a five year period because of intolerable symptoms. Medically treated patients with triple vessel disease and impaired LV function fare less well, with an annual mortality of up to 10%. Operative mortality for these patients is approximately 2%.

4. *Left main stem disease*

   Patients with left main stem disease treated medically have a five year survival of 65%, compared with 85% if they are treated with surgery. Although LV dysfunction, increasing age, systemic hypertension, left dominance and additional coronary artery lesions increase the operative risk, recent reports indicate that the early mortality has fallen from 4% to <2% in this group.

5. *Unstable angina*

The patient with unstable angina is best treated with maximal medical thereapy (see Ch. 1), and subsequently investigated by elective coronary arteriography one week after relief of symptoms. Intra-aortic balloon counterpulsation may control angina refractory to medical treatment. In a small proportion of patients symptoms cannot be adequately controlled despite maximum medical treatment and in this subgroup urgent coronary arteriography is required. This may reveal a lesion suitable for thrombolysis or PTCA. Occasionally, emergency CABG will be necessary.

Elective CABG in the patient with unstable angina is associated with a 3% early mortality which may approach 5% if emergency operation is necessary. Although five year survival is similar in medical and surgical groups, 30–40% of patients will cross over the surgical group during follow-up.

6. *Acute myocardial infarction*

Facilities for emergency revascularisation in patients with evolving myocardial infarction are not generally available. In the single centre with a large experience of this technique, early mortality was reduced by early intervention (revascularisation complete by six hours of the onset of chest pain). As expected, patients with diffuse disease and cardiogenic shock fare less well.

Relief of symptoms with surgery

Following CABG, 75–90% of patients note symptomatic improvement, and 35–55% of patients become pain free. 5–6% are symptomatically worse after operation. Patients who are completely revascularised achieve a better result, as do patients with a short history, those with current or recent employment, strong motivation and *typical* angina. Patients with atypical chest pain and/or breathlessness obtain less benefit.

Symptomatic improvement is related to graft patency (see p. 64). Angina recurs at a rate of 3–4% per annum and at 11 years only 30% of patients are symptom free.

Surgical risk factors

1. *Age*

Operative mortality is increased, and five year survival is reduced in patients over 65 years of age. Factors such as left main stem disease and LV dysfunction are particularly poorly tolerated in the elderly and may increase the operative mortality three or four fold. Although improved myocardial preservation has reduced the risk of operation in this age group, the operative mortality for patients over 75 years of age remains at 5–10%. Duration of hospital stay is also significantly longer in elderly patients.

2. *Sex*

   Women have a higher operative mortality (×2), a higher incidence of preoperative infarction and a less favourable prognosis than men after CABG. Left coronary ostial stenosis also appears more common in women. When results are normalised for body surface area the differences between men and women are less striking.

3. *Diabetes mellitus*

   Patients with diabetes have more diffuse disease and a higher incidence of other risk factors (e.g. hyperlipidaemia, systemic hypertension, LV disease) than the general population. Postoperative renal dysfunction and wound infection are also more common in diabetics.

   Operative mortality for diabetics is twice that for non-diabetics, but whether the diabetes is controlled by diet and oral hypoglycaemics or insulin appears to make little difference. Five year survival is also worse for diabetics than non-diabetics (77–80% vs 88% respectively).

4. *Left ventricular dysfunction*

   Abnormal LV function increases both the early and late mortality from CABG. However, improvement in myocardial protection has meant that patients who would not previously have been considered for CABG on the grounds of poor LV function, now undergo operation with an acceptable mortality. Few patients have such poor LV function that they are not surgical candidates, but it should be remembered that symptomatic improvement after CABG is poor in patients in whom breathlessness was the major preoperative symptom.

5. *Additional procedures*

   In most centres additional procedures (e.g. aortic or mitral valve replacement, excision of LV aneurysm) significantly increase the mortality of CABG alone.

Surgical technique

Details of the surgical technique are beyond the scope of this book. The principle of surgical treatment is to attempt to revascularise all major coronary arteries having a significant stenosis (>50% obstruction of the lumen), whilst protecting the myocardium from ischaemic damage during the procedure. This is achieved on cardiopulmonary bypass using systemic and topical cooling, together with cold potassium cardioplegia.

Coronary artery bypass grafting using reversed lengths of saphenous vein may be combined with excision of myocardial scar, resection of an LV aneurysm or mitral valve replacement if appropriate.

Endarterectomy, particularly of the right coronary artery, allows CABG to be undertaken on vessels that would normally be unsuitable for grafting. Early experience indicated that endarterectomy was associated with a high (15–16%) peroperative infarction rate, but with the advent of cardioplegia this has fallen to 4–5% (i.e. twice the observed rate in patients without endarterectomy). Perhaps surprisingly, patency rates are similar in right coronary grafts that have had an associated endarterectomy when compared with those that have not.

Recent evidence suggests that the internal mammary (IMA) graft to the left anterior descending and/or the right coronary artery has superior patency to vein grafting. Although the vessel is frequently small, and additional expertise and time are necessary to harvest the vessel and complete the anastomosis, graft flow is adequate and graft atherosclerosis is uncommon. IMA grafts are particularly useful for the patient with diffuse LAD disease, or when the saphenous vein is unsuitable for grafting. IMA graft harvesting is time consuming and therefore unsuitable for emergency operations and in the elderly where the duration of the operation is important.

Complications

1. *Death*

   Overall operative mortality from series of unselected patients is 1–2% for males and 4–5% for females. Important determinants of operative mortality include the experience of the surgical team, age and sex of the patient, and if surgery is undertaken as an emergency.

   In recent series (since 1979), left main stem disease and LV dysfunction have ceased to be operative risk factors. Improved survival can be attributed to a number of factors including better preoperative care and stabilisation of the patient, improved anaesthesia and haemodynamic monitoring and more thorough myocardial protection — this is despite the patient poulation undergoing CABG becoming older and technically more demanding.

2. *Preoperative infarction*

   Use of cold potassium cardioplegia has reduced the risk of preoperative infarction to 2–8%. Risk factors responsible for operative mortality do not contribute to the preoperative infarction rate. Furthermore, preoperative infarction has little detrimental effect on long-term mortality.

3. *Arrhythmias*

   Supraventricular and, less commonly, ventricular arrhythmias occur in 10–30% of patients following CABG. Hypokalaemia and arterial hypoxaemia frequently contribute to the incidence of arrhythmias. Small doses of beta blockers (e.g. metoprolol 50 mg or propranolol 40 mg twice daily) are usually effective, and prophylaxis may be appropriate in the early postoperative period. Haemodynamic compromise may require urgent DC countershock (40 joules).

4. *Cerebral dysfunction*
   Cerebral complications affect up to 2% of patients, and are more frequent in the elderly. In approximately 50% of these patients the neurological disturbance is transient, with no residual sequelae.

5. *Wound infection*
   Infection involving the sternotomy or leg wounds may be troublesome and mar an otherwise successful operation. Deep infection leading to sternal instability, osteomyelitis, or mediastinitis is rare. Very occasionally skin grafting may be required to the leg.

GRAFT PATENCY AND OCCLUSION

A number of factors influence graft patency rates. Surgical technique (including the proximal and distal anastomosis, length of graft, and preservation of the vein endothelium), arterial runoff and the administration preoperative antiplatelet drugs are all important determinants. Occlusion rates vary between 2% and 5% per annum, and occlusion due to poor surgical technique most commonly occurs in the first few months after operation. Strictures related to the proximal anastomosis are seen more frequently, and graft flows of <50 ml/min are associated with a higher incidence of occlusion.

More rapid progression of coronary atherosclerosis in grafted native vessels compared with ungrafted vessels has been noted in some patients. Progression of disease proximal to the anastomosis is common and may eventually cause complete occlusion of the native vessel.

Two pathological processes may be seen in vein grafts and contribute to poor function. Diffuse or segmental intimal fibrous hyperplasia is a non-progressive condition which may develop within the first year. Vein atherosclerosis is a progressive disease, and by 10 years 50% of vein grafts show some degree of atherosclerosis and 30–40% are occluded. Patency rates are higher in sequential and 'Y' grafts due to the higher flow rates. Hyperlipidaemia (especially low HDL and high LDL) is an important contributor to graft occlusion.

Reoperation

With increasing numbers of patients undergoing CABG more patients will come to reoperation. Currently the reoperation rate in various series is 6–17% or 0.5% of patients/annum. Since the late 1970s the aim of the initial operation has been complete myocardial revascularisation (i.e. more grafts); this being the case, the major indication for reoperation is graft occlusion rather than progress of disease in the native circulation.

Risk factors for patients undergoing reoperation are similar to patients having their first operation with the exception that diabetes mellitus is twice as common in those undergoing a second procedure (i.e. 20% vs 10%). Operative mortality for reoperation has decreased due to improved myocardial preservation from 10% to 2–5%. Patients with the highest mortality include the elderly, those with incomplete initial revascularisation or left main stem disease. Overall, the preoperative infarction rate for reoperation is approximately 5%. Only 50% of patients obtain symptomatic relief five years after reoperation, compared with 60–70% following the initial procedure. Not surprisingly graft patency rates are a little lower than for the first operation.

Rehabilitation and return to work

In an uncomplicated case, discharge from hospital can be expected on the seventh to tenth postoperative day. Ideally, structured rehabilitation classes are commenced prior to discharge and continued as an outpatient (as in the survivors of acute myocardial infarction, see Ch. 2). Not only is camaraderie between patients who have undergone the same procedure helpful in restoring confidence, but the rate of progress can be individually tailored to the requirements of a particular patient. Education regarding modification in the lifestyle of the patient (e.g. smoking, obesity, stress etc.) may also be undertaken at this time.

Likelihood of return to work after CABG is a complex subject. Although symptoms are improved in up to 90% of patients, only half of these patients return to work. Return to work is related to socioeconomic status, as well as the length of time the patient has been off work. Favourable factors determining return to work include short duration of illness, young age (<55 years), high income, and a good symptomatic result. Inappropriate advice from physicians, and lack of understanding from employers are major contributors to the low rate of return to work.

4. SYSTEMIC HYPERTENSION

In the United Kingdom at least 10% of the adult population has a significant elevation in systemic blood pressure (>160/95) which is 'essential' (primary or idiopathic) in 90–95% of cases and 'secondary' in the remainder. It has been shown conclusively that a reduction in blood pressure in the patient with moderate/severe hypertension (>115 mmHg diastolic) improves prognosis and reduces the risk of target organ damage (cardiac, cerebral, and renal disease). Furthermore, a number of clinical trials indicate that the treatment of lesser degrees of hypertension (90–105 mmHg diastolic) is beneficial in terms of prognosis and complications, but against this must be balanced the problems of treating a frequently asymptomatic individual for the remainder of his life with drugs that have potential side effects for a marginal improvement in longevity.

There is no simple answer as to how thoroughly the patient with elevated blood pressure should be investigated nor at what level of blood pressure should treatment begin. Blood pressure is distributed as a continuous variable within the population, it increases with age and the risks from hypertension are proportional to the absolute level of both systolic and diastolic blood pressure. Hypertension in the patient less than 40 years of age warrants full investigation (see p. 71), but the recent increase in concern over cost effectiveness, the low yield from expensive (and unpleasant) investigations, and the reduction in enthusiasm for the surgical treatment of some forms of secondary hypertension, has led many to treat hypertension without extensive investigation. Indeed, it has been estimated that <5% of patients with hypertension are treated by hospitals and that the remainder are treated by general practitioners in the community with little or no prior investigation.

Most would agree that a sustained blood pressure of 160/100 or more warrants treatment, and that lesser degrees of hypertension should be treated in the younger patient, in those who are pregnant, in association with aortic dissection, or if there is evidence of target organ damage (e.g. history of transient ischaemic attacks, an abnormal electrocardiogram or renal impairment).

PATHOPHYSIOLOGY OF ESSENTIAL HYPERTENSION

Although the pathophysiology of 'essential' systemic hypertension is ill understood it is clear that the aetiology is multifactorial. Factors responsible for maintaining the blood pressure within the normal fine limits include the control of extravascular fluid volume by hormones (renin, antidiuretic hormone, sex hormoens, ?natriuretic hormone), neural mechanisms (inlcuding the autonomic and central nervous systems) and other agents that influence arterial tone and reactivity (e.g. prostacyclin and vasoactive amines) against a background of inherited predisposition and environmental influences (e.g. stress and urban living).

AETIOLOGY

Some of the more frequent causes of systemic hypertension are listed in Table 4.1.

SYMPTOMS

Only if the patient has severe hypertension is he symptomatic from the elevation in blood pressure per se. This group of patients experience headaches which may have the features of elevated intracranial pressure, namely, increased severity in the mornings and on lying down and exacerbation by coughing, laughing and straining. There may also be symptoms from target organ damage and in certain forms of secondary hypertension an elevation in blood pressure is associated with a symptom complex (listed below).

Table 4.1 Causes of systemic hypertension

1. Essential hypertension (95%)
2. Secondary hypertension (5%)
   a. Renovascular disease (fibrous dysplasia, atherosclerosis, trauma)
   b. Renal parenchymal disease (including glomerulonephritis, interstitial nephritis, pyelonephritis, diabetes, gout, analgesic nephropathy, amyloid, collagen vascular disease, obstructive uropathy)
   c. Coarctation of the aorta
   d. Adrenal disease (primary hyperaldosteronism, phaeochromocytoma, Cushing's syndrome, congenital adrenal hyperplasia)
   e. Other hormonal causes (carcinoid, acromegaly, phaeochromocytoma [extra adrenal in 10%])
   f. Drugs (oral contraceptives, corticosteroids, liquorice, carbenoxolone sodium, non-steroidal anti-inflammatory agents, MAOIs, sympathomimetics)
   g. Hypertension of pregnancy (including pre-eclampsia)
   h. Neurogenic hypertension (raised intracranial pressure, tetanus, bulbar poliomyelitis)
   i. Other causes (including acute intermittent porphyria, lead poisoning)

Symptoms from target organ damage

1. *Cardiac*
   Angina, palpitations, dyspnoea, orthopnoea, nocturnal dyspnoea, nocturia
2. *Cerebral*
   Cerebrovascular events, transient ischaemic attacks, visual disturbance, headache, hypertensive encephalopathy (which see)
3. *Renal*
   Anorexia, nausea, vomiting, polyuria, fluid retention, symptoms related to anaemia
4. *Peripheral vascular disease*
   Claudication

Symptoms associated with secondary hypertension

1. *Primary hyperaldosteronism*
   Symptoms related to hypokalaemia, namely thirst, polyuria, cramps, muscle weakness, paralysis, tetany
2. *Phaeochromocytoma*
   Paroxysmal headaches, sweating, palpitations, anxiety, tremor, chest and abdominal pain, prostration and weight loss
3. *Carcinoid syndrome*
   Flushing, telangiectasia, diarrhoea, tricuspid regurgitation and pulmonary stenosis. Transient systemic hypertension rarely occurs but sustained hypertension is not a feature of carcinoid syndrome

In addition to enquiring into possible symptoms associated with hypertension, a detailed drug history should be taken (including oral contraceptives, liquorice, carbenoxolone sodium and analgesic abuse). A positive family history of cardiac, cerebral, renal, endocrine disease or systemic hypertension may also be important.

CLINICAL EXAMINATION

1. *Measuring the blood pressure*
   Physicians trained in the United Kingdom are usually taught to take the diastolic pressure as the point at which the sounds become muffled (Korotkoff 4th phase), rather than when the sounds disappear (5th phase). In the USA and in epidemiological studies the 5th phase is frequently used. In the normal adult the 4th and 5th phases are closely related (within 5 mmHg) but in certain conditions (e.g. aortic regurgitation) the 5th phase is unrecordable. The 5th phase

more closely approximates to the diastolic pressure measured from an intra-arterial catheter. A useful approach is to record both phases at each patient visit (e.g. 160/100/95). Care must be taken to properly apply the appropriate sized cuff so that the bladder overlies the brachial artery. A casual single recording is related to prognosis in untreated hypertension but it is customary to take three or four readings before labelling a patient as 'hypertensive'. If the initial reading is elevated the blood pressure should be recorded again at the end of the examination when the patient is more relaxed. To dismiss an elevated blood pressure as being related to anxiety is inappropriate as it is likely that the patient who is anxious in the clinic will be anxious on other occasions in the course of a normal day with an associated elevation in blood pressure. If coarctation of the aorta is a possibility then the blood pressure should be recorded in both arms and in the legs as well in order to confirm the diagnosis and localise the site of the coarctation.

In clinical studies observer error and bias are reduced by means of sphygmomanometers in which the actual value cannot be read until the reading has been taken. This avoids the temptation of rounding the reading up or down to the nearest 5 or 10 mmHg.

2. *Examination of the optic fundi*

Examination of the optic fundi gives the unique opportunity of directly observing structural changes in central arteries and veins. It is often assumed that the Keith-Wagener classification of vascular changes within the fundus refers exclusively to changes brought about by systemic hypertension. However the early grades of retinopathy (I & II) can equally well be due to arteriosclerotic disease which normally accompanies the ageing process.

Grade I: Increased light reflex from arteries ('copper-wiring'), segmental irregularity in calibre of arteries, or diffuse narrowing which increases the normal vein: artery ratio of 3:2.

Grade II: Arterial sclerosis and medial hypertrophy give rise to apparent venous 'kinking' followed by arterio-venous 'nicking'. This phenomenon occurs because the artery and vein share a common adventitial sheath at the point of cross-over and the hypertrophied artery compresses the thin walled vein.

Grade III: Haemorrhages and exudates. Haemorrhages result from leaking capillaries, and their shape is determined by the layer in which they occur.

'Flame' shaped lesions lie superficially in the nerve fibre layer of the retina and 'blot' haemorrhages lie between the bipolar nuclei. The 'dot' lesions associated with diabetic retinopathy represent microaneurysms. 'Cotton wool' exudates are areas of focal ischaemia caused by micro-infarction in the nerve fibre layer of the retina. Choroidal infarcts and serous retinal detachment may occasionally occur.

Grade IV: Papilloedema is characterised by loss of the physiological 'cup' (usually 2 dioptres in depth), the disc margin becomes pink and blurred (which is more marked on the nasal aspect) and the retinal veins are engorged. Papilloedema also occurs in other circumstances including raised intracranial pressure, retinal vein thrombosis and retrobulbar neuritis.

Survival of patients with untreated hypertension is related to the appearance of the fundi ranging from 85% for Grade I to <5% for Grade IV at 5 years. Examination of the fundi is a useful means of assessing the length of time the blood pressure has been elevated in the patient who presents with severe hypertension for the first time. Florid changes of hypertensive retinopathy are rarely seen in the elderly. Arterial tortuosity may be particularly marked in adults with coarctation of the aorta.

3. *Cardiovascular system*

Other than the elevation in blood pressure, there may be clinical evidence of hypertensive heart disease or peripheral vascular disease. The arterial pulse has a full volume and normal upstroke. In peripheral vascular disease the lower limb pulses may be reduced or absent and bruits may be audible over the abdominal aorta, femoral or popliteal vessels. Both carotid arteries should be palpated individually and carefully examined for bruits. The apex beat is sustained in left ventricular hypertrophy. On auscultation the first heart sound is normal, A2 may be accentuated and in cases of severe left ventricular disease or left bundle branch block (in which left ventricular ejection is prolonged), splitting of the second sound is paradoxical. A systolic ejection click may be heard, and a fourth (atrial) sound is frequently audible. In more severe disease a third heart sound and pulmonary oedema may be evident.

4. *Examination of the abdomen*

Enlarged kidneys may be palpated (e.g. in polycystic disease), and loin tenderness suggests renal tract infection.

Renal bruits (from renal artery lesions) are often very difficult to detect.

5. *Other features*
The general appearance of the patient may indicate the underlying diagnosis, particularly in cases of hypertension associated with endocrine disease (e.g. Cushings syndrome, acromegaly).

INVESTIGATIONS

1. Screening investigations for all patients
   a. Haematology: full blood count, ESR
   b. Biochemistry: electrolytes, urea, uric acid, liver function tests, calcium, fasting glucose and lipids
   c. Urinalysis: 'stick' testing (blood, protein, glucose), microscopy (cells, microorganisms, casts), culture
   d. Chest radiograph (PA)
   e. Electrocardiogram (12 lead)
2. Further investigations for selected patients
   a. Intravenous urography (including rapid sequence films). An IVU is reserved for patients younger than 40 years, or when there are other reasons to believe renal disease is a factor in the hypertension
   b. Renin and aldosterone assays
   c. Adrenaline, noradrenaline, metadrenaline, normetadrenaline, vanillylmandelic acid (VMA) assays
   d. Abdominal CT
   e. Renal scanning (^{99m}Tc-DTPA, ^{99m}Tc-DMSA)
   f. Renal digital vascular imaging (DVI)
   f. Renal arteriography
   h. Adrenal scanning (^{131}I-cholesterol or ^{75}Se-methylcholesterol)
   i. Adrenal venous sampling

Investigation and treatment in selected causes of secondary hypertension

a. Renovascular disease
Sudden onset of severe systemic hypertension resistant to conventional therapy in young females, men in late middle age, or following trauma, may be the result of unilateral renovascular disease. Clinical suspicion may be increased by the presence of an abdominal bruit and severe hypertensive retinopathy. Renovascular disease accounts for 3–6% of cases of hypertension in most series, but this figure falls to approximately

1% in an unselected population. The aetiology of the arterial lesion may be congenital or acquired; however the mechanism of blood pressure increase is similar in all forms of renovascular hypertension, namely vasoconstriction mediated by renin release from the ischaemic kidney stimulating the renin-angiotensin system.

Fibrous dysplasia

Seen predominately in females aged 20–50 years, accounting for 30% of all cases of renal artery stenosis. Affects the distal two thirds of the main renal arteries, and branch arteries are involved in up to 10% of cases. A number of variants have been described involving one or more layers of the artery, but fibromuscular (medial) dysplasia is the most common. Aneurysmal dilatation occurs as a result of the connective tissue abnormality and other major vessels (e.g. carotid and mesenteric arteries) may also be affected. Renovascular hypertension is also seen in children due to congenital renal artery dysplasia and occasionally as a result of renal artery thrombosis following umbilical artery catheterisation.

Atherosclerosis

Occurs in men over the age of 50 years usually in association with widespread arterial disease. Diabetes mellitus is also more common in this group. In contrast to fibrous dysplasia the proximal third of the renal artery is diseased. Renal artery thrombosis on an atherosclerotic plaque or dissection may result in sudden severe hypertensiosn.

Investigation

Intravenous urography with rapid sequence films is the initial investigation of choice. Exposures are taken immediately after injection of contrast and at 1 minute intervals until 5 minutes and then at 15 and 30 minutes. The triad of disparity in renal size (>1.5 cm), delay in the appearance of the nephrogram (>1 minute after the normal side) and late increase in density of the nephrogram on the affected side will identify 80–90% of patients. Occlusion of the artery will be detected in >95% of cases. The addition of renal scanning with ^{99m}Tc-DTPA or ^{99m}Tc-DMSA not only improves the sensitivity and specificity of the diagnosis when used in combination with urography, but further information regarding the contribution of each kidney to overall renal function is made available. More recently, digital vascular imaging (DVI) has allowed the renal arteries to be assessed in some detail using a peripheral venous injection, and this technique may become the procedure of choice for screening patients with suspected renal artery stenosis. Prior to surgical intervention or angioplasty, the detailed anatomy of the renal arteries needs to be defined by arteriography. Selective renal arteriograms are taken as well as an abdominal aortogram via a percutaneous (Seldinger) approach from the femoral artery. The outcome of surgery cannot necessarily be predicted from the appearance of the arterial lesion(s) demonstrated by arteriography. Renal vein sampling is frequently combined with arteriography; if the renal vein renin ratio is >1.5–2.0:1 then the results of operation are more favourable. These investigations are best carried out in a specialist unit as false values may be obtained if the catheterisation technique is not meticulous. Although 25% of patients have bilateral disease, one side usually predominates and unilateral renal ischaemia is responsible for the hypertension in these patients. Estimations of peripheral vein renin has no place in the assessment of renovascular disease, but angiotensin antagonists (e.g. captopril) may have a role in predicting the outcome of surgery. Split renal function studies (with selective catheterisation of each ureter) are now rarely performed as nuclear studies give similar information non-invasively.

Treatment
Initial enthusiasm for the surgical approach to renovascular hypertension has been tempered by only moderate success (approximately 50%) in terms of blood pressure control in the majority of patients together with an early surgical mortality of 5–15% even in specialised units. In particular, middle-aged and elderly patients with a generalised arteriopathy do poorly. However, in the young patient with fibrous dysplasia in whom unilateral renal ischaemia has been clearly documented the results can be excellent. Emphasis of surgical treatment is on renal artery reconstruction and conservation of renal tissue rather than nephrectomy. Patients with a short history do better than those with chronic elevation in blood pressure as levels of renin have often fallen to normal in the latter group. Balloon dilatation of arterial lesions by percutaneous angioplasty offers promise in selected patients.

With the advent of oral angiotensin converting enzyme inhibitors the medical control of blood pressure has become easier in patients unsuitable for surgery (see p. 85).

2. Coarctation of the aorta
Most cases of coarctation of the aorta present in infancy with left ventricular failure associated with poor peripheral pulses in which case surgical correction is undertaken between 1 and 5 years of age. A proportion of patients remain undetected until adolescence or middle age when they are found to have systemic hypertension, left ventricular failure, or present following aortic rupture or dissection or after a cerebral haemorrhage secondary to rupture of an aneurysm of the circle of Willis. It is uncommon for a patient with untreated coarctation to live to more than 50 years of age.

In adults, the coarctation is seen as a discrete infolding of the aortic wall which narrows the lumen just distal to the ligamentum arteriosum. Coarctation of the aorta accounts for approximately 8% of congenital heart disease in infants, 4.5% in children, and 8% of congenital heart disease presenting for the first time in adults. Males are affected more frequently than females (3:1), and there may be associated abnormalities (VSD, PDA, tubular hypoplasia of the aortic arch, mitral valve anomalies) and a bicuspid aortic valve occurs in 50% of patients. 45% of patients with Turner's (XO) syndrome have coarctation of the aorta. Infective endocarditis may occur usually in association with a bicuspid aortic valve.

In the adult, symptoms may be inconspicuous and an elevated blood pressure is found as an incidental finding. Alternatively, the patient may complain of undue fatigue, non-specific chest pain, headaches, or intermittent claudication. Clinical examination reveals a muscular torso and upper limbs and rather underdeveloped lower limbs. Collateral vessels may be visible and can be palpated over the scapular region, the neck and the anterior chest wall. Upper limb and carotid pulses have a full volume and sharp upstroke. Simultaneous palpation of the radial and femoral pulses reveals the femoral pulses to be absent, or delayed with respect to the radial pulses (radiofemoral delay). A systolic ejection click indicates an additional bicuspid aortic valve and bruits may be audible from collateral vessels over the anterior chest wall and scapulae.

Investigation

The classic radiographic findings of coarctation of the aorta are obscuring of the aortic knob and rib notching. Normally, the aortic knob is discrete and represents the aorta just distal to the left subclavian artery. In coarctation a 'figure three' configuration is seen in the left superior mediastinum composed of the dilated left subclavian artery and post-stenotic dilatation of the descending aorta separated by an indentation, the coarctation. Rib notching is indicative of erosion of bone by dilated intercostal vessels which act as part of the collateral supply to the distal aorta. Notching of the undersides of the ribs is associated with a rim of sclerotic bone which helps differentiate pathological notching from normal rib irregularities. Only 75% of patients with coarctation have rib notching; furthermore rib notching can be seen in the absence of coarctation, but in these cases the notching is more medial. The electrocardiogram may show non-specific features of left ventricular hypertrophy on voltage criteria and a 'strain' pattern. Coarctation of the aorta and associated abnormalities can be demonstrated by cross-sectional echocardiography from the suprasternal notch. Although high quality images can be obtained in infants and children, adequate visualisation may be difficult in adults. Coarctation can also be demonstrated by thoracic CT, but contrast aortography remains the definitive investigation. A 7F or 8F pigtail catheter is introduced via the right brachial artery and advanced to the left ventricle. Pressures are recorded within the left ventricle and across the outflow tract to exclude additional outflow tract obstruction. If a gradient is demonstrated, cineangiograms are recorded in the long axial and apical four chamber views to profile the outflow tract and to exclude an associated VSD. If there is evidence of aortic valve disease an ascending aortogram is recorded in the left anterior oblique projection. The catheter is then advanced down the descending aorta. In severe coarctation it may be impossible to pass the catheter past the site of the narrowing, but in minor degrees of coarctation a withdrawal gradient can be recorded between descending aorta and the aortic arch at the level of the left subclavian artery. A further aortogram is recorded at the level of the right subclavian artery in the AP projection. In addition to the site of the coarctation, anomalies of the head and neck vessels and the extent of the collateral vessels are visible.

Treatment

Surgical resection is undertaken with an end-to-end anastomosis, but if the ends of the aorta cannot be approximated it may be necessary to interpose a short Dacron conduit. The early mortality is 0–2%. Major complications include paraplegia secondary to ischaemia of the spinal cord and necrotising mesenteric arteritis. Rebound hypertension may occur in the immediate postoperative period. Many adults who have undergone successful correction of a coarctation have persistent hypertension following operation or an abnormal blood pressure response to exercise. Life expectency is reduced despite surgical intervention.

3. Primary hyperaldosteronism (Conn's syndrome)

An aldosterone secreting adenoma accounts for 70% and adrenal hyperplasia (zona glomerulosa) for approximately 20% of cases of primary hyperaldosteronism. Some patients have the typical biochemical findings with no detectable adrenal abnormality. The relationship of this group to patients with low renin 'essential' hypertension is unclear. A high serum sodium (>142 mmol/l) is associated with hypokalaemia (<2.7 mmol) and a metabolic alkalosis (HCO_3 >33 mmol). In hypertensive patients the most common cause of this combination of biochemical abnormalities is diuretic therapy although the alkalosis is usually less marked and the blood urea may be slightly elevated on diuretics. Regional assays of renin and aldosterone have simplified diagnosis. In primary hyperaldosteronism an elevated aldosterone level unresponsive to a high sodium diet (200–300 mmol/day), is associated with a low plasma renin unresponsive to a low sodium diet (10–20 mmol/day). The biochemical abnormalities are more marked in the patient with an adenoma (frequently female) than in patients with adrenal hyperplasia.

Investigation

Rational treatment can only be planned following the accurate localisation of an adenoma or identification of bilateral adrenal hyperplasia. Adrenal venography is technically difficult but may show a unilateral increase in adrenal vein aldosterone in the presence of an adenoma. Hyperplasia may be identified by abdominal CT and/or ultrasound but adenomas are usually too small to visualise. Adrenal scanning using ^{131}I-cholesterol or ^{75}Se-methylcholesterol can detect an adenoma as small as 0.5 cm diameter. Arteriography and retroperitoneal air insufflation are unreliable.

Treatment

Surgical removal of the adenoma results in an increase in the serum potassium in most cases and correction of the hypertension in approximately 50% of patients. Transient postoperative salt depletion may require oral 9alpha-fludrocortisone or parenteral DOCA. In cases of bilateral adrenal hyperplasia the biochemical abnormalities and hypertension are treated with aldosterone antagonists (e.g. spironolactone 100–800 mg daily or amiloride 10–40 mg daily).

The appropriate investigation and management of these patients should be managed in a specialised centre.

4. Phaeochromocytoma

Phaeochromocytomas are catecholamine secreting tumours that develop from chromaffin cells. Most are solitary adrenal tumours, 10% are malignant and 10% are bilateral. Extra adrenal tumours, which account for 10% of the total, are known as paraganglionomas or chemodectomas if they arise in chemoreceptor tissue. Of the extra adrenal tumours most are found in the abdomen usually at the aortic bifurcation (Organ of Zuckerkandle).

Investigation

Assays of urinary normetanephrine and metanephrine are the most sensitive indicators of a phaeochromocytoma and are least affected by antihypertensive drugs (e.g. clonidine, methyldopa), or certain foodstuffs (e.g. bananas, coffee). Urinary vanillylmandelic acid (VMA) should also be measured and more recently plasma radioimmunoassays (using catechol O-methyl transferase) have become more generally available. The role of plasma as opposed to urinary assays has not been clarified. Repeated estimations may be necessary and samples taken immediately after a hypertensive attack are more likely to be positive. A spectrum of catecholamines can be excreted by the tumour; an excess of adrenaline may indicate an extra adrenal site and a high secretion of dopamine suggests malignancy. Urine collections should be kept refrigerated and acidified (pH<3.5) and plasma samples must be drawn from an indwelling venous cannula so that the patient is in a basal unstressed state during sampling.

Localisation of the tumour is essential prior to surgical exploration. A combination of abdominal CT, ultrasound, and ^{131}I meta-iodobenzylguanidine (^{131}I MIBG) scanning will localise most tumours. Intravenous urography and nephrotomograms may also be required but iodine containing contrast media (e.g. Conray) may itself increase levels of metanephrine. Venous sampling and aortography should only be undertaken with prior alpha and beta blockade. Alpha blockade is established with phenoxybenzamine and subsequently beta blockade is added to the drug regimen. Beta blocking drugs must not be given to the patient prior to alpha blockade as serious hypertension may develop from the unopposed actions of the circulating catecholamines. Titration of the individual drugs is more satisfactory than administration of a combination preparation (e.g. Labetalol). An echocardiogram should also be recorded as 50% of patients who die from phaeochromocytoma have myocardial disease secondary to catecholamine overactivity.

Treatment

Surgical removal with prior alpha and beta blockade is curative in most patients. In cases of malignant disease or where removal is incomplete the blood pressure can be controlled by drug therapy. An alternative approach is to reduce synthesis of noradrenaline and adrenaline by inhibiting the hydroxylation of tyrosine to dopa using alpha-methyl-p-tyrosine (Alpha-MT).

Associated diseases

1. Phaeochromocytoma and medullary carcinoma of the thyroid (Sipple's syndrome). Inherited (autosomal dominant) in 5% of cases. Other hormones (e.g. ACTH, serotonin) may also be produced.
2. Neurofibromatosis. Occurs in 5% of patients with phaeochromocytoma.
3. Cerebellar haemangioblastoma (von Hippel-Lindau syndrome) is rarely associated with phaeochromocytoma.

5. Cushing's syndrome

Moderate (rarely severe) systemic hypertension is present in 80% of patients with Cushing's syndrome. 60–70% of these cases are due to an excess of ACTH from a pituitary source, usually an adenoma, stimulating cortisol release from the adrenal cortex. The exact mechanism of the hypertension is unclear but it appears not to be related to the severity of the biochemical abnormality; aldosterone and the renin-angiotension system as well as cortisol excess have been implicated.

Investigation

The clinical appearance of the patient may make the diagnosis obvious, namely centrally obese with thin limbs, muscle wasting, osteoporosis, thin papery skin, bruising etc. The detailed investigation of these patients is beyond the scope of this book but includes a dexamethasone suppression test, ACTH assay and estimation of urinary free cortisol.

Treatment

Patients with a pituitary adenoma are treated with trans-sphenoidal hypophysectomy or irradiation, and those with a solitary adrenal adenoma by unilateral adrenalectomy. Cytotoxic drug therapy may be required in cases of adrenal carcinoma.

6. Hypertension associated with oral contraceptives

Approximately 5% of patients taking combination oral contraceptives develop a significant elevation in systemic blood pressure. In most cases the increase in blood pressure is only moderate, but accelerated hypertension with renal impairment has been reported. In those who are susceptible blood pressure increases progressively from the first year of use. High blood pressure is seen more frequently in patients over 35 years, in those with a family history of hypertension, and in patients who have been hypertensive during a previous pregnancy. Discontinuing the preparation results in normalisation of blood pressure within a few months in most cases but some patients appear to develop 'essential' hypertension in later life.

Oestrogens have been implicated by their salt retaining action via the renin-angiotensin system, but hypertension can occur in patients on progesterone-only preparations. It is advisable for patients with pre-existing hypertension to use an alternative form of contraception.

8. Hypertension of pregnancy (see Ch. 18)

TREATMENT OF SYSTEMIC HYPERTENSION

Most studies show that the quality of life in the patient with undiagnosed hypertension is similar to normal controls. This is an important consideration in both the diagnosis and treatment of a patient with hypertension. Not only may the patient feel subjectively less well once he has been 'labelled' hypertensive but side effects from the medication may compound the problem.

Several general principles apply once the decision has been made to treat the blood pressure:

1. Explain fully the necessity of treating the blood pressure, even if the patient is asymptomatic (target organ damage etc). Counselling by the clinic nurse may be particularly helpful as the patient is more likely to discuss minor difficulties with the treatment.
2. Ideally, a once or twice daily regimen is chosen for better patient compliance. 50% of patients on long-term antihypertensive therapy do not comply with instructions and this may lead to the false assumption that the blood pressure is 'resistant' to conventional therapy.
3. A combination of two agents in low dose may be synergistic rather than additive (e.g. diuretic + beta blocker) and associated with less side effects than a larger dose of a single agent. If the dose of a drug needs increasing, tablet strength should be increased rather than tablet numbers. Two drugs combined in one tablet (e.g. Dyazide) is more acceptable to the patient, although scientifically less acceptable to the clinical pharmacologist.
4. Minor adjustments to therapy (e.g. timing of doses of diuretics or beta blockers) in individual patients should be undertaken to minimise side effects and a prior explanation that alterations will be necessary is worthwhile.

Non-drug treatment

Behavioural modification although good in principle is often difficult to achieve. Minor reductions in blood pressure can result from meditation and biofeedback in some individuals, but the sustained reduction of blood pressure by these techniques is probably not possible in most patients. Obesity should be avoided but the assessment of a reduction in blood pressure as a result of weight loss alone is complicated by the changes in blood pressure brought about by changes in the cirumference of the arm. A standard cuff applied to an obese arm tends to overestimate the blood pressure. Patients should be advised not to smoke and to take regular exercise. However, there is no clear evidence that the latter has a beneficial effect on blood pressure. A no-added salt diet (<150 mmol/day) with additional diuretics is more palatable than a low or no salt diet.

Drug treatment

A 'stepped-care' approach is used most frequently in the control of elevated blood pressure. That is, one, two or three drugs are used in combination until the blood pressure is adequately controlled. A satisfactory antihypertensive regimen should be uncomplicated, well tolerated and inexpensive, leading to smooth control of both systolic and diastolic blood pressure. Until recently, a diuretic was chosen as the initial treatment for most patients, followed by the addition of a beta blocker. This combination restores the blood pressure to acceptable levels in 80% of patients. However, it has become apparent that the side effects from diuretics may equal or exceed those from beta blockers (particularly in men), and this coupled with the possible 'protective' effects of beta blockade in coronary artery disease make beta blockers the first line of treatment for most patients. The addition of a vasodilator controls the blood pressure in a further 10–15% of patients and in the remaining 5–10% (who frequently have renal impairment), the blood pressure is difficult to control. Except in accelerated hypertension (see p. 87) there is little place for inpatient management of hypertension unless metabolic disturbances (e.g. renal impairment) are a cause for concern. Admitting the patient to hospital encourages inactivity and removes him from his normal environment.

Beta blockers

The mode of action of beta blocking agents in systemic hypertension is incompletely understood. After commencing therapy there is an initial 15–20% fall in cardiac output due both to a slowing in heart rate and a reduction in contractility. Within a few weeks the cardiac output returns to normal despite continuing blood pressure control. Changes in heart rate and cardiac output may precede the reduction in blood pressure. Plasma renin activity is reduced by the $beta_2$ effect of beta blocking drugs which inhibits renal renin release. Although patients with 'high' renin hypertension respond well to beta blockade, 'low' renin hypertension may be controlled equally well; furthermore, the adequacy of blood pressure control is not related to the fall in plasma renin activity brought about by beta blockade. Despite the fall in blood pressure systemic vascular resistance may actually increase early after commencing therapy due to unopposed alpha activity; subsequently the peripheral resistance falls to normal or low levels. Beta blockers also have actions on the central nervous system, autoregulation, baroreceptors and catecholamine biosynthesis.

Choice of beta blocker

The present choice of nine types of oral and seven intravenous preparations of beta blocking agents available in the UK (Table 4.2; see also Ch. 1, Table 1.8) appears excessive. However, the differing characteristics of the various preparations in terms of half-life, selectivity and lipid solubility are important factors in choosing the appropriate drug for a particular patient. The antihypertensive action of the various beta blockers is similar but the tolerance in terms of side effects varies from patient to patient.

Propranolol, the original beta blocker, blocks the action of both myocardial (beta$_1$) and peripheral (beta$_2$) receptors. Blocking of bronchial beta$_2$ receptors may precipitate acute airflow obstruction in the form of bronchial asthma in susceptible individuals; even in patients who experience no respiratory symptoms subtle changes in airway resistance may be detectable on formal respiratory function tests. Another important complication of non-selective agents is exacerbation of intermittent claudication from peripheral vascular disease (which frequently accompanies systemic hypertension and coronary artery disease). Unopposed alpha adrenergic activity on peripheral smooth muscle when beta$_2$ receptors are blocked may also result in cool extremities and Raynaud's phenomenon. Propranolol also suffers from extensive (up to 70%) first pass metabolism, which may vary depending on liver function. In addition, hepatic metabolites (e.g. 4-hydroxy-propranolol) may have activity that differs from the parent compound, and this causes the duration of therapeutic activity to exceed the plasma half-life. Hepatic metabolism probably accounts for the very variable doses of propranolol (up to 4 g daily) necessary for blood pressure control in some individuals. This is not true for some of the newer preparations (e.g. Atenolol) in which the dose response curve is flat, and therefore more convenient.

More recent 'cardioselective' preparations (e.g. Atenolol, Metoprolol, Acebutolol) primarily block beta$_1$ actions but increasing doses may also

Table 4.2 Beta-blocking drugs available in the UK

	Oral preparation	Intravenous preparation	Beta$_1$ selectivity	Once daily preparation
Propranolol	+	+	−	+
Oxprenolol	+	+	−	+
Nadolol	+	−	−	+
Acebutolol	+	+	−/+	−
Sotalol	+	−	−	−
Timolol	+	−	−	−
Metoprolol	+	+	+	+
Atenolol	+	+	+	+
Pindolol	+	−	−	−
Practolol	−	+	+	−

block beta$_2$ receptors; furthermore, the dose at which a 'selective' agent becomes non-selective varies from patient to patient. Other important secondary properties of beta blocking drugs include differences in protein binding and lipid solubility. Agents that have low lipid solubility are less affected by hepatic metabolism, tend to have a longer half-life, and cross the blood-brain barrier less readily. Central nervous system side effects are seen less frequently with these compounds. Some beta blocking drugs, particularly Pindolol, possess beta agonist activity (intrinsic sympathomimetic activity or ISA) which is thought to be beneficial in certain circumstances. Pindolol is said to reduce contractility and pulse rate less than other beta blockers without ISA and ISA may result in less airflow obstruction and lower limb ischaemia. Selectivity is more important property than ISA in this regard. Membrane stabilising activity (MSA) or the local anaesthetic action of certain beta blockers (e.g. Oxprenolol) is of no clinical consequence.

Side effects

In 5–10% of patients undesirable side effects either prevent beta blocking drugs from being used for the control of systemic hypertension or necessitate a reduction in drug dosage. More frequently encountered side-effects are listed in Table 4.3.

Diuretics

The mode of action of diuretics is ill understood. Initially, there is a slight increase in systemic vascular resistance associated with a fall in plasma volume, extracellular fluid volume and cardiac output. After 6–8 weeks systemic vascular resistance falls perhaps due to a direct vasodilator action of the drug itself despite an increase in plasma renin activity. The secondary fall in blood pressure may be due to changes in vascular reactivity or a re-setting of autoregulatory responses, and is probably not related to salt balance because aldosterone secretion via the

Table 4.3 Side-effects of beta blocking drugs

Cardiovascular
Low cardiac output, sinus bradycardia, atrioventricular block, systemic hypotension, ?exacerbate coronary artery 'spasm', precipitate myocardial ischaemia following acute withdrawal. Cool extremities, exacerbate peripheral vascular disease, Raynaud's phenomenon. Muscle fatigue, reduced exercise tolerance

Pulmonary
Exacerbate airflow obstruction (bronchial asthma, obstructive bronchitis, emphysema)

Gastrointestinal
Anorexia, nausea, diarrhoea

Central nervous system
Depression, insomnia, vivid dreams, hallucinations, impaired concentration, drowsiness, impotence

Metabolic
Hyperlipidaemia ($\uparrow$ triglyceride, $\uparrow$ VLDL, $\downarrow$ HDL), potentiate hypoglycaemia

Skin
Rash, oculomucocutaneous (rash, dry eyes, sclerosing peritonitis)

renin-angiotensin system causes a reduction in sodium excretion. Renal blood flow actually increases after 8 weeks diuretic therapy. Diuretics (particularly thiazides) work poorly when the creatinine clearance falls below 20 ml/min. Furthermore, diuretic therapy for the hypertensive patient with severe renal impairment may be detrimental as renal perfusion falls and renin levels increase still further.

1. *Thiazides*

Thiazides inhibit sodium reabsorption in the ascending limb of the loop of Henle and the distal convoluted tubule. Recent data indicate that intolerance to diuretics may be more common than previously reported particularly in men. There is little to choose between the numerous thiazide diuretics available, therefore one of the cheaper preparations should be used (e.g. Bendrofluazide). Most thiazides are effective within 2 hours of oral ingestion. Little evidence exists to suggest that a long-acting preparation is superior to those with a short duration of action, except for the convenience of a more controlled diuresis (which in hypertension is unimpressive after the first few weeks of therapy anyway). Thiazide diuretics have a flat dose response curve and the minimal effective dose should be used whenever possible. Metolazone has a similar site of action to thiazides including some proximal tubular activity and may offer advantages over thiazides in that it continues to be active in patients with renal impairment.

Side effects of thiazide include impotence and loss of libido, diarrhoea, tinnitus, hypokalaemia, glucose intolerance, hyperuricaemia, disturbances of the lipid profile and hypercalcaemia.

a. *Hypokalaemia*

Most patients on thiazide diuretics show a small reduction in serum potassium but little or no change in total body potassium. Potassium supplements need not routinely be given unless the patient is symptomatic (e.g. cramps, muscle weakness, fatigue), being treated for fluid retention or receiving concomitant digoxin therapy. Small doses of potassium incorporated into some thiazides (e.g. 8 mmol K^+ per Navidrex K tablet) do little to offset hypokalaemia. If necessary, potassium chloride (approximately 80 mmol/day) is used as a supplement because the chloride helps in the correction of the metabolic alkalosis as well as the hypokalaemia. A more reasonable approach is to use a combination diuretic that includes a potassium sparing preparation (e.g. Amiloride, Triamterene) although significant hypokalaemia can still occur. Additional prerenal azotaemia may result from over vigorous diuresis and hyponatraemia can occur in a setting of renal impairment with tubular damage.

b. *Glucose intolerance*
Reversible impairment of glucose tolerance may accompany treatment with thiazides. Raised insulin levels probably indicate impaired peripheral utilization of insulin and concomitant hypokalaemia may be a related factor. Frank diabetes indicates a pre-existing diabetic tendency and patients with known diabetes may require an adjustment of their hypoglycaemic agents. Whether long-term thiazide therapy can actualaly lead to the development of diabetes in a previously normal patient is uncertain.

c. *Hyperuricaemia*
An elevation in uric acid as a consequence of untreated hypertension may be compounded by treatment with thiazide diuretics. Acute gout or gouty nephropathy is rare, and as in hyperuricaemia from other causes, the level at which asymptomatic hyperuricaemia should be treated is variable. Although the first uricosuric diuretic (tienilic acid) was withdrawn from the market because of toxicity, more will become available in due course. A tendency to hyperuricaemia may be compounded by the addition of a beta blocking drug.

d. *Lipid abnormalities*
An inconsistent increase in plasma triglyceride and/or cholesterol levels has been reported in association with thiazide therapy; the long-term implications with regard to the development of atherosclerosis have yet to be determined.

e. *Hypercalcaemia*
A small rise in serum calcium due to increased tubular reabsorption of calcium and potentiation of the renal action parathyroid hormone is only important in patients who have a primary abnormality of parathyroid function or are taking vitamin D preparations in which case thiazides are contraindicated.

f. *Hypomagnesaemia*
Chronic diuretic ingestion causes magnesium depletion, and occasionally frank hypomagnesaemia, which can result in cardiac arrhythmias (classically atypical ventricular tachycardia or Torsade de pointes, see Ch. 16) and an increased risk of digoxin toxicity.

g. *Other side-effects*
Hypersensitivity reactions include skin rashes, vasculitis, thrombocytopaenic and non-thrombocytopaenic purpura, glomerulonephritis, pancreatitis and hepatic dysfunction.

2. *Loop diuretics*

This group of drugs inhibit sodium reabsorption in the ascending limb of the loop of Henle. In patients with normal renal function, thiazides are more potent than loop diuretics in controlling hypertension. Loop diuretics (frusemide, bumetanide and ethacrynic acid) are appropriate for the patient with fluid retention, or renal impairment (serum creatinine >200 μmol/l, creatinine clearance <25 ml/min).

3. *Potassium sparing diuretics*

These drugs act on the distal convoluted tubule and early collecting duct to block sodium-potassium exchange either by a direct action (amiloride and triamterene) or as a result of aldosterone antagonism (spironolactone). Given alone their antihypertensive actions are weak but they are useful if given in combination with thiazides (e.g. Moduretic, Dyazide) as they prevent hypokalaemia and alkalosis. Spironolactone can be used in the treatment of primary hyperaldosteronism (Conn's syndrome) but the onset of action is delayed for 2–4 days and it may be poorly tolerated due to gynaecomastia or menstrual disturbances. Amiloride is a reasonable alternative. This group of drugs should be used with care in patients with renal impairment as they may result in hyperkalaemia.

Vasodilators

The vasodilators act either predominately on the venous capacitance vessels or the arterial resistance vessels (see Ch. 7). They are particularly useful when used in patients with renal impairment, in combination with other agents and in patients with airflow obstruction.

1. *Hydrallazine*

Side effects prevent the use of hydrallazine as a single antihypertensive agent but in combination with a diuretic and beta blocker adequate blood pressure control is achieved in most patients. Initially a small dose (e.g. 25 mg twice daily) should be added to the regimen and gradually increased to a maximum of 200 mg daily in divided doses. Hydrallazine reduces systemic vascular resistance by a direct action on arteriolar smooth muscle with little associated effect on the venous capacitance vessels. Increase renin activity and fluid retention can be counteracted by the beta blocker and diuretic respectively. First pass metabolism is mainly via acetylation in the liver and a larger dose will be required for a comparable haemodynamic effect in fast acetylators. Hydrallazine metabolites are excreted in the urine and plasma levels of the parent compound are not related to therapeutic activity.

Most of the side-effects (e.g. tachycardia, flushing, headache) occur when the drug is used alone. Cardiac work may increase and this can occasionally precipitate angina.

Drug induced lupus occurs with increasing frequency in doses over 200 mg daily (depending on acetylator status) and although this is nearly always reversible it may persist. Tachyphylaxis is a problem, particularly when the drug is used as a vasodilator in heart failure.

2. *Minoxidil*

This drug acts in a similar manner to hydrallazine and therefore also needs to be given in combination due to side effects of fluid retention and tachycardia. It is a powerful long-acting vasodilator and is useful in renal failure. Profuse (reversible) hair growth precludes treatment in many patients particularly females. An initial once daily dose of 5 mg increasing to 50 mg daily is used in most patients.

3. *Prazosin*

Although originally introduced as a peripheral vasodilator it is now clear that prazosin is a post ganglionic $alpha_1$ receptor blocker thereby preventing noradrenaline binding to the smooth muscle cell. It acts both as an arteriolar and venodilator, cardiac output changes little and renal blood flow is not impaired. Prazosin can be ued as a single antihypertensive agent because the preservation of $alpha_2$ activity prevents reflex tachycardia and renin release. The drug is well absorbed orally and although the plasma half-life is 3–4 hours the therapeutic activity lasts considerably longer such that twice (or three times) daily dosing is adequate for most patients.

The 'first-dose phenomenon' resulting in severe hypotension or loss of consciousness shortly after ingesting the first tablet is particularly common in patients on large doses of diuretics or other vasodilators. In order to avoid this side effect, a very small test dose (0.5 mg) should be taken lying down last thing at night. Similar symptoms after the first dose are very rare. Prazosin is well tolerated in most patients. Side-effects include headaches, lack of energy, sexual and bladder dysfunction and nasal congestion. Postural hypotension may occur in the elderly, and rare reports of a positive antinuclear factor have been reported.

4. *Angiotensin converting enzyme inhibitors*

Angiotensin II, the most powerful naturally occurring vasoconstrictor, is generated from the action of angiotensin converting enzyme (ACE) or Kininase II on the substrate angiotensin I. ACE, which is found mostly in the lung, has other important actions including an effect on noradrenaline release at nerve endings and an inhibitory action on the vasodilator bradykinin. Orally available ACE inhibitors include Captopril, and more recently Enalapril (which is said to be less toxic). Secondary actions of ACE inhibitors include competitive inhibition of angiotensin II at the receptor site. They are very effective antihypertensive agents particularly in patients with renal disease; although they are more potent in high renin hypertension they may also be used in low renin hypertension.

A 'first dose phenomenon' may occur if the patient is taking large doses of diuretics, therefore a small (6.25 mg) test dose should be given initially and then cautiously increased to a maximum of 150 mg three times daily. Numerous side effects reported early in the clinical experience of the drug were related to the high doses initially suggested by the manufacturer. Most of the more troublesome side effects are related to the sulfhydryl group which is absent in the newer compound Enalpril. Minor side-effects include a metallic taste in the mouth, pruritis, fever and skin rash. Agranulocytosis, proteinuria and membranous nephropathy are rarely encountered. Renal complication can be precipitated in patients with a low cardiac and poor renal perfusion. Requirements for diuretics are reduced due to a reduction in aldosterone and hyperkalaemia may occur by the same mechanism.

5. *Calcium channel blockers*

This group of drugs (nifedipine, diltiazem and verapamil) has been widely used in the treatment of angina and is a useful addition to the available antihypertensive agents. They cause a reduction in systemic vascular resistance by arteriolar vasodilatation and may be used alone as there is no reflex tachycardia. Side effects include facial flushing and fluid retention. Depression of atrioventricular node conduction varies between drugs (see Ch. 1, Table 1.10), but combinations of calcium antagonists and beta blockers have been found to be effective in hypertension without untoward side-effects.

Other drugs

1. *Methyldopa*

This drug is used less frequently for the treatment of hypertension because of intolerable side-effects particularly in men. The metabolite of methyldopa, alphamethyl-noradrenaline, acts centrally by stimulating post-synaptic alpha$_2$ receptors which inhibit sympathetic outflow from the central nervous system and reduce peripheral arterial resistance. Common side effects include sedation, bad dreams, depression, dry mouth and sexual dysfunction. A positive direct Coombs test occurs in 20% of patients but haemolytic anaemia is rare (<1%). Less common side-effects include fever, hepatitis, myocarditis, eosinophilia and a positive antinuclear factor.

2. *Clonidine*

The central action of clonidine is similar to methyldopa but the drug is better tolerated; the drug may also have a peripheral action on smooth muscle. Like methyldopa, levels of renin are reduced, but it acts equally well in low renin hypertension. The major problem with clonidine, which has also been reported with methyldopa, is a rebound phenomenon which occurs following the abrupt withdrawal of the drug. This resembles the symptoms of a phaeo-chromocytoma, namely headaches, anxiety, sweating and severe hypertension associated with increased levels of catecholamines. Reinstitution of clonidine is effective treatment but intravenous phentolamine may rarely be necessary. This side-effect may be troublesome in the elderly who forget to take their medication.

3. *Adrenergic neurone blockers*

Ganglion blocking drugs (Debrisoquine, Bethanidine and Guanethidine) are rarely used today because of side-effects, particularly exercise and orthostatic hypotension, failure to ejaculate and interaction with tricyclic antidepressants. However, a number of patients have been taking these preparations for many years with no apparent ill effect.

ACCELERATED HYPERTENSION

A fuller understanding of the pathophysiology of accelerated hypertension and the appreciation of the concept of cerebral autoregulation has led to more rational treatment of accelerated (or 'malignant') hypertension. In the past, inappropriate enthusiasm for the aggressive treatment of accelerated hypertension frequently resulted in catastrophic cerebral or myocardial dysfunction.

Within certain limits of pressure cerebral perfusion is regulated by the appropriate vasoconstriction or dilatation of cerebral vessels in order to maintain cerebral perfusion constant despite variations in systemic pressure. A breakdown in this mechanism may result in spasm of the intracerebral vessels, cerebral oedema, intracerebral haemorrhage and lacunar infarction. In the patient with long-standing systemic hypertension thickened cerebral vessels are better able to tolerate high extremes of pressure; satisfactory autoregulation in this group probably occurs between a mean arterial pressure of 90–180 mmHg. However, the patient with no previous history of hypertension may experience a breakdown in autoregulation at a mean arterial pressure as low as 120 mmHg. It is this group who present with accelerated hypertension and in most cases the blood pressure is relatively easy to control.

Features of accelerated hypertension

Accelerated hypertension is said to occur in approximately 1% of patients with systemic hypertension. Although the full syndrome of accelerated hypertension with hypertensive encephalopathy is rare in clinical practice one or more of the following features may be present:

1. Elevated systemic blood pressure (usually >120 mean)
2. Proteinuria, haematuria, renal impairment
3. Third heart sound, acute pulmonary oedema
4. Hypertensive retinopathy (haemorrhages, exudates, papilloedema)
5. Confusion, headache, change in conscious level, visual disturbance, neurological deficit, seizures
6. Microangiopathic haemolytic anaemia, disseminated intravascular coagulopathy.

Without appropriate treatment death results from cerebrovascular events, renal failure or acute myocardial infarction. If left untreated, 20% of patients are alive after one year and 1% after 5 years.

Treatment

The aim of treatment is to reduce the blood pressure to normal levels over a 6–24 hour period depending on the condition of the patient. A reasonable approach is to commence oral treatment with a combination of a beta blocker and diuretic. If renal impairment is present, a loop diuretic may be more appropriate than a thiazide (*NB*: large doses of diuretics are not usually required). To this is added hydrallazine 10–20 mg given intramuscularly as necessary. This regimen results in a gradual reduction in blood pressure and can be administered by a nurse. As the oral agents begin to work, the doses of intramuscular hydrallazine required will become less frequent. Subsequently, the dose of the beta-blocker can be increased and an oral vasodilator (hydrallazine, prazosin, captopril) can be increased as necessary. Alternatively, hydrallazine can be given intravenously (5–10 mg).

A number of other agents may be useful in the management of accelerated hypertension:

1. *Nitroprusside*
   This intravenous arterial and venodilator is a potent antihypertensive agent and has the advantage of a short half-life of 1–3 minutes. It should be used in an ICU environment (see p. 134) but with experience it is a safe and predictable drug. If used long-term the accumulation of thiocyanate may be a problem and this should be monitored. As a vasodilator, it is particularly useful in the patient with hypertensive left ventricular disease and pulmonary oedema.

2. *Diazoxide*
   Initial use of this drug suggested that it should be

administered as a rapid intravenous bolus of 150 or 300 mg in order to saturate protein binding sites. As a consequence of this approach sudden uncontrolled hypotension resulted in a number of instances of stroke and acute myocardial infarction. A constant infusion of 5–30 mg/min diazoxide provides a smoother reduction in blood pressure and is a more appropriate method of administration. The absence of venodilator activity may result in a reflex tachycardia, increased cardiac output and fluid retention. Long-term oral therapy with diazoxide is poorly tolerated because of gastrointestinal side-effects and glucose intolerance.

3. *Labetolol*

This drug is a combination of a non-selective beta blocker and a weak alpha blocker. It is effective as an intravenous infusion (commencing at 2 mg/min). The alpha action brings about an early reduction in blood pressure and beta blockade inhibits renin activity. Side effects include postural hypotension, gastrointestinal disturbances, depression, and occasional formation of antinuclear and antimitochondrial antibodies of uncertain significance.

4. *Other drugs*

Intravenous methyldopa (400–1000 mg over 20 minutes) and intravenous clonidine (300 µg over 10 minutes) have also been advocated for the treatment of accelerated hypertension.

All patients being treated for accelerated hypertension should be managed with an intravenous line in situ so that inadvertent hypotension can be corrected with intravenous fluids; furthermore, potent short-acting drugs like nitoprusside are more easily controlled with an indwelling arterial line (see Ch. 20).

5. PULMONARY OEDEMA

PHYSIOLOGY

The symptoms, signs and radiological features of acute pulmonary oedema occur as a result of an abnormal increase in extravascular lung water. The forces relating the movement of water across the pulmonary vascular bed are summarised by Starling's Law:

$$Q = KS \left[(P_{CAP} - P_{IS}) - (\pi_{CAP} - \pi_{IS}) \right]$$

Where: Q = net transvascular flow
K = filtration coefficient
S = capillary surface area
P_{CAP} = pulmonary capillary hydrostatic pressure
P_{IS} = pulmonary interstitial pressure
π_{CAP} = capillary oncotic pressure
π_{IS} = interstitial oncotic pressure

In health, Q is >1, favouring the egress of fluid from capillaries into the interstitium, which is returned to the circulation via an efficient system of lymphatic drainage. Thus, major factors controlling the accumulation of extravascular fluid include changes in capillary permeability (K), capillary hydrostatic pressure (P_{CAP} and capillary oncotic pressure (π_{CAP}). In conditions in which there is a chronic elevation in capillary hydrostatic pressure, lymphatic flow may increase twenty-fold thereby preventing the accumulation of interstitial fluid.

Pulmonary oedema represents the response of the lung to a physiological insult, and should not in itself be thought of as a primary diagnosis. Similarly, the term 'left ventricular failure' and 'congestive cardiac failure' are best avoided. Frequently the patient said to be 'left ventricular failure' may not have significant left ventricular dysfunction (e.g. in isolated mitral stenosis). Furthermore the term 'congestive cardiac failure' is used by some to mean acute pulmonary oedema, whereas others take it to mean fluid retention, or alternatively right ventricular dysfunction secondary to left-sided disease. In most patients, acute pulmonary oedema has a cardiac basis and the capillary hydrostatic pressure (P_{CAP}), measured at the bedside as the pulmonary arterial capillary wedge pressure (PACWP), is >12 mmHg; in other patients the major abnormality involves the alveolar-capillary membane (non-cardiac pulmonary oedema).

Causes of pulmonary oedema are listed in Table 5.1.

SYMPTOMS

1. *Dyspnoea*

   Acute shortness of breath, described by the patient as 'choking', 'drowning' or 'suffocation', is characteristic of pulmonary oedema. Typically, the patient is anxious and frightened, and the release of endogenous catecholamines may provoke subendocardial ischaemia, impede left ventricular filling and exacerbate the haemodynamic disturbance. There may be no previous history of similar episodes, particularly if the attack is associated with a change in heart rhythm (as in mitral stenosis) or acute myocardial infarction (which may be painless). If there is only a modest increase in PACWP at rest (12–15 mmHg), the patient may

Table 5.1 Causes of pulmonary oedema

1. Pulmonary venous hypertension
   Left ventricular disease (elevated LVEDP)
   Mitral valve disease (mitral stenosis and/or regurgitation)
   Pulmonary veno-occlusive disease
2. Reduced intrathoracic (interstitial) pressure
   Removal of a pleural effusion
   Drainage of a pneumothorax
3. Decreased plasma oncotic pressure*
4. Altered alveolar-capillary membrane
   Infections (bacterial including legionella, viral, parasitic)
   Inhaled toxins (smoke, chlorine, elevated FIO_2)
   Non-thoracic trauma (including burns)
   Gastric aspiration
   Uraemia
   Pulmonary contusion
   Pulmonary embolism (including air and amniotic fluid)
   Near drowning
   Massive transfusion of blood products (unfiltered)
   Disseminated intravascular coagulation
   Acute radiation pneumonitis
   Hypersensitivity pneumonitis (Busulphan, Nitrofurantoin, Methotrexate)
5. Lymphatic disorder
   Lymphangitis carcinomatosis
   'Reimplantation syndrome' (following lung and heart-lung transplantation)
   Fibrosing lymphangitis
6. Other causes (aetiology unclear)
   High altitude
   'Neurogenic'
   Narcotic abuse ('Heroin lung')
   Post cardiopulmonary bypass or haemodialysis

* There is debate as to whether a low serum albumin per se results in pulmonary oedema.

only complain of shortness of breath during exertion due to further elevation of the PACWP in association with an increase in cardiac output. Wheezing may be prominent in acute pulmonary oedema and the possibility of airflow obstruction must always be excluded.

Shortness of breath is a non-specific symptom and occurs in many other conditions including:
a. Pulmonary disease
    Airflow obstruction, restrictive lung disease, infection, pneumothorax, pulmonary collapse, pleural effusion, upper airway obstruction
b. Pulmonary embolism and thromboembolic disease
c. Primary pulmonary hypertension
d. Aortic dissection
e. Acidosis (hyperventilation)
f. Anaemia
g. Anxiety
h. Pregnancy

2. *Orthopnoea*
    When the patient lies flat, systemic venous return and pulmonary capillary hydrostatic pressure increase and vital capacity is reduced. Thus, pulmonary compliance is reduced, the work of breathing increases and a sensation of dyspnoea is apparent. Patients with chronic airflow obstruction may also experience orthopnoea due to the accumulation of secretions and difficulties in expectorating when recumbent. Rarely, orthopnoea is the presenting symptom in certain neurological conditions (e.g. myasthaenia gravis, motor neurone disease) in which diaphragmatic function is abnormal.

3. *Cough*
    Prior to the onset of paroxysmal effort dyspnoea, nocturnal coughing may be the only symptom of an elevated PACWP. Nocturnal coughing (±wheezing) is also a feature of bronchial asthma. A non-productive cough which may be exercise related also occurs in patients with pulmonary hypertension from other causes (e.g. primary pulmonary hypertension, Eisenmenger's syndrome).

4. *Paroxysmal nocturnal dyspnoea*
    Sudden awakening from sleep with severe shortness of breath is a feature of acute pulmonary oedema and bronchial asthma. Both may be associated with coughing; in pulmonary oedema the sputum is copious, frothy and blood-stained, whereas in bronchial asthma the sputum is tenacious and may contain plugs laden with eosinophils (Charcot-Leiden crystals). Formerly, massive haemoptysis (pulmonary apoplexy) frequently accompanied severe mitral stenosis but

this is now rare. The patient may sit on the edge of the bed gasping for breath ('air hunger'), or pace around the room and open the window. The attack may subside without specific treatment, and in the asthmatic patient self-administered bronchodilators by inhaler are frequently rapidly effective.

PHYSICAL SIGNS

1. *Low cardiac output ('shock')*
   Sweating, restlessness and confusion are associated with a low cardiac output. Poor peripheral perfusion results in muscle fatigue and cool extremities. Endogenous catecholamine release causes a sinus tachycardia with an elevation in systemic blood pressure. However, a raised blood pressure per se is rarely a cause of acute pulmonary oedema unless there is concomitant left ventricular disease. Careful examination of the fundi will reveal hypertensive retinopathy if previously elevated blood pressure was significant. Low cardiac output or 'shock' is also a feature of aortic dissection, occult blood loss and tension pneumothorax.

2. *Cyanosis*
   Central cyanosis is apparent when there is 5 g or more of reduced haemoglobin per 100 ml blood. Assuming a normal haemoglobin concentration, cyanosis is visible when the PaO_2 is <8.0 kPa (60 mmHg). In pulmonary oedema, reduced oxygenation results from an increase in right to left shunting secondary to V/Q mismatch.

3. *Auscultation of the heart*
   The cause of the pulmonary oedema may become obvious following auscultation of the heart. The loud S1, opening snap and mid-diastolic murmur of mitral stenosis, the single S2 and ejection systolic murmur of aortic stenosis, or the loud pansystolic murmur of mitral regurgitation. One of the earliest and most sensitive indicators of left ventricular dysfunction is a ventricular diastolic gallop or third heart sound (S3). This is a low-pitched sound, best heard with the bell of the stethoscope and localised to the apical region. It occurs 140–160 ms after S2, and coincides with the rapid filling wave of the apexcardiogram. An S3 may be the only clinical evidence of ischaemic heart disease, and in the presence of pulmonary oedema is easily overlooked. In young patients an S3 is 'physiological', but this finding is rare after 40 years of age. In addition, an atrial gallop (S4) may be appreciated at the lower left sternal border or medial to the

apical impulse. An S4 is rarely a normal finding, but it occurs in a number of conditions including left ventricular disease (due to cardiomopathy or ischaemia), systemic hypertension or aortic stenosis.

4. *Auscultation of the lungs*

Late (end) inspiratory crackles audible over the lung bases are characteristic of pulmonary oedema. Crackles are short, explosive, discontinuous sounds of variable intensity generated by the sequential opening of small airways at varying lung volumes and transpulmonary pressures. In the presence of peribronchial oedema, airway opening during inspiration is delayed. Indeed, the lung volumes at which airway opening begins may exceed functional residual capacity (FRC), such that during tidal respiration some alveoli are never ventilated; this results in V/Q mismatch, right to left shunting and arterial hypoxaemia. Crackles are poorly transmitted and are not audible at the mouth. However, in the late stages of pulmonary oedema (alveolar flooding, Table 5.2), inspiratory and expiratory rattles can be heard throughout the airways and are frequently audible from the bedside. Late inspiratory crackles also occur in fibrosing alveolitis. The findings in chronic airflow obstruction differ in that the crackles are early in inspiration or expiratory, they are scanty and low pitched, and are transmitted to the mouth. Wheezes may be prominent in acute pulmonary oedema, particularly in the smoker with previous airflow obstruction.

5. *Other findings*

Pulsus paradoxus and pulsus alternans may occur in association with acute pulmonary oedema.

INVESTIGATIONS

1. *Chest radiograph*

Chest radiography is the single most important investigation in the patient with acute pulmonary oedema. A high quality PA film may be difficult to obtain if the condition of the patient is poor, but a PA film taken with the patient sitting on the edge of the bed is a reasonable compromise. Accurate assessment of the heart size and superior mediastinum is not possible on a portable AP film. It should be emphasised that the timing of clinical events and abnormalities seen on the chest radiograph do not necessarily coincide. Mild elevation of PACWP (12–15 mmHg) may be undetectable on the chest radiograph, similarly the patient who has been adequately treated with a diuretic or vasodilator therapy may still have radiological evidence of pulmonary oedema despite the PACWP having returned to normal (<12 mmHg). Table 5.2 indicates the stages of pulmonary oedema, the radiological findings and the corresponding levels of PACWP.

Long-standing elevation of PACWP (e.g. in chronic mitral valve disease) may be associated with pulmonary haemosiderosis and rarely pulmonary ossification. Haemosiderin deposits are found mainly in the air spaces and within the lymphatics and arise as a result of microvascular bleeding.

Definitions

a. *Kerley B lines*

Thin, dense horizontal lines (<2 mm wide and <3 cm long) which lie perpendicular to the pleural surface and are best seen in the lower lobes. These peripheral lung markings are due to fluid (fibrosis or tumour) within the interlobular septae.

b. *Kerley A lines*

Longer straight or oblique lines in the upper lobes running from the periphery to the hilum of the lung.

c. *Kerley C lines*

Network of Kerley B lines forming a 'spiders web' in the lower lobes.

Pleural effusions (if present) are more common on the right side. Subpleural collections of fluid mimic elevation of the diaphragm, and accumulation of fluid within the interlobar spaces may simulate a tumour (pseudotumour) on the PA film. The proximal pulmonary arteries are prominent if the PA pressure exceeds 50 mmHg. In dilated cardiomyopathy the heart is enlarged, but the heart size may be normal in

Table 5.2 Manifestations of acute pulmonary oedema

Stage	Physiology	Radiology	PACWP (mmHg)
I	Increase in transpulmonary flow from intravascular to interstitial compartment. Increased lymphatic flow	Redistribution. Upper lobe blood diversion	12–15
II	Lymphatic capacity exceeded. Fluid accumulates around bronchioles and arterioles (loose interstitial spaces)	Perivascular and interstitial oedema. Interlobar fluid. Subpleural effusions	18–25
IIIA	Tight interstitial space and early alveolar oedema		
IIIB	Alveolar flooding (air space oedema). Alveolar-capillary disruption. Increase in permeability of alveolar-capillary membrane	Perihilar haze. 'Butterfly' or 'bats wing' distribution	>25

Table 5.3 Pulmonary oedema with a small heart (CTR <0.55)

1. Acute myocardial infarction
2. Mitral stenosis
3. Acute mitral regurgitation (chordal or papillary muscle rupture)
4. Aortic stenosis
5. Acute aortic regurgitation
6. Hypertrophic cardiomyopathy
7. Restrictive cardiomyopathy
8. Constrictive pericarditis
9. Adult respiratory distress syndrome (ARDS)

many other cardiac causes of acute pulmonary oedema (Table 5.3).

2. *Electrocardiogram*

Most patients with acute pulmonary oedema have an abnormal electrocardiogram. Changes typical of acute myocardial infarction may be apparent, but if the history is short the ECG may be entirely normal. Poor anterior R wave progression is a non-specific indicator of left ventricular disease. Long-standing systemic hypertension may cause increased voltages and repolarisation changes. A rapid ventricular rate in atrial fibrillation may be enough to provoke pulmonary oedema in the previously fit patient with moderate mitral stenosis.

3. *Echocardiography*

This is a useful investigation once the patient has recovered from the acute attack. Abnormalities of segmental wall motion are seen in myocardial infarction and left ventricular aneurysms may be visualized. Other forms of myocardial disease (e.g. dilated cardiomyopathy) and valvular heart disease may also be identified by echocardiography.

4. *Arterial blood gases*

Increased right to left shunting due to V/Q mismatch results in arterial hypoxaemia. Hyperventilation causes a low $PaCO_2$. If sequential blood gas estimations indicate a rising $PaCO_2$ the patient may be tiring (Type II respiratory failure) and in need of mechanical ventilation; alternatively, the patient may have additional airflow obstruction and have been given too high a concentration of oxygen (hence removing 'hypoxic drive'), or excessive doses of opiates. A low pH and HCO_3 indicate a metabolic acidosis.

MANAGEMENT

Acute pulmonary oedema is a medical emergency and in the majority of patients it will respond rapidly to the appropriate medication. When the patient is first seen, a large bore (16 or 18G) peripheral venous line is inserted for access, and blood drawn for routine testing including electrolytes, urea, creatinine, cardiac enzymes, haemoglobin and white cell count. If the expertise is available, a central venous line is preferable but not mandatory. If the patient fails to respond to initial treatment and requires vasodilator therapy, a radial arterial line and Swan-Ganz balloon flotation catheter (see Ch. 20) are used to optimise 'preload' and 'afterload'. As a general principle, all drugs should be administered by the intravenous route because of the unreliability of perfusion and tissue absorption from alternative sites. Digoxin in particular should never be given by intramuscular injection as it is tissue bound, and absorption is erratic even when the injection site is well perfused.

Initial treatment

1. *Diuretics*

   In the patient who has not received regular diuretics, Frusemide 40 mg IV is an adequate initial dose. Larger doses may cause electrolyte imbalance (hypokalaemia) and intravascular fluid depletion. Increased doses of loop diuretics may be required in patients taking diuretics chronically, or those with renal impairment. Following the administration of frusemide an improvement in the condition of the patient may be noted within a few minutes, prior to the onset of a diuresis. This is due to the secondary weak venodilator property of frusemide. If loop diuretics fail to provide an adequate diuresis, then Dopamine at a renal dose $(2-4\mu g/kg/min)$ should be added to the regimen.

2. *Opiates*

   The role of opiates in acute pulmonary oedema is threefold. Fear and anxiety are alleviated, endogenous catecholamine drive is reduced, and opiates are also venodilators. Diamorphine 2.5–5.0 mg IV has the disadvantage that it has to be reconstituted prior to administration, but the euphoriant effect is superior to Morphine 5.0–10.0 mg IV (which is a satisfactory alternative). An anti-emetic is administered as a routine (e.g. Metoclopramide 10 mg IV, Prochlorperazine 12.5 mg IV) because excessive vagal activity is undesirable. Care is taken not to overdose the patient who may have additional airflow obstruction, and Naloxone (Narcan) 3 mg IV should be available if respiratory depression ensues.

3. *Oxygen*

   An attempt is made to maintain the PaO_2 >8 kPa (60 mmHg) by enriching the inspired air. It is difficult to achieve an FIO_2 >0.6–0.7 without intubation and mechanical ventilation, but adequate oxygenation can be achieved in most patients by means of an MC mask or 60% Ventimask.

Nasal cannulae or 'prongs' are more comfortable, but the delivered oxygen concentration is variable. All inspired gas should be humidified. If adequate oxygenation cannot be maintained, the patient will require mechanical ventilation ($\pm$PEEP).

4. *Aminophylline*

Aminophylline is particularly useful in the patient in whom wheezing is a manifestation of pulmonary oedema, or when there is additional airflow obstruction. Not only does aminophylline relax bronchial muscle, but it also possesses actions as a mild diuretic, a weak venodilator and a cardiac stimulant. Unwanted side effects include central nervous stimulation, headaches, flushing, tremors, nausea and palpitations. Uncontrolled vasodilatation may result in systemic hypotension. An initial dose of 5 mg/kg as an IV infusion over 15 minutes, is followed by a constant infusion of 0.9 mg/kg/h, which is adjusted to maintain the serum level at 10–20 mg/l.

5. *Nitrates*

This group of vasodilators act mainly on the venous circulation to cause a reduction in 'preload' (see Ch. 7). In addition, inappropriate systemic hypertension can be controlled and there may be a direct vasodilator action on the coronary circulation. With experience this group of drugs are not difficult to use, but should only be given in an ICU setting (with monitoring of systemic arterial, PA and PACWP) when administered by the IV route.

A number of preparations are available including:

a. Nitroglycerine (Nitrocine) 50 mg/50 ml 5% Dextrose @ 20–25 μg/min.

b. Isosorbide Dinitrite (Cedocard, Isoket) 10 mg/100 ml 5% Dextrose @ 2–10 mg/h (33–167 μg/min).

6. *Arterial vasodilators*

These drugs are used to reduce systemic vascular resistance (arterial impedance) or 'afterload' and hence cardiac work (see Ch. 7). Like nitrates they have a short half life and are administered by a continuous IV infusion in an ICU environment. Frequently a combination of arterial and venous dilators is used to provide optimum loading conditions.

Arterial vasodilators include:

a. Sodium Nitroprusside (Nipride) 50 mg/500 ml 5% Dextrose @ 0.5–8.0 μg/kg/min.

b. Salbutamol (Ventolin) 5 mg/500 ml 5% Dextrose @ 3–20 μg/min.

c. Phentolamine (Rogitine) 50 mg/500 ml 5% Dextrose @ 0.1–2.0 mg/min.

7. *Digoxin*

There is no place for the use of digoxin in the management of the patient in acute pulmonary oedema unless the attack has been precipitated by atrial fibrillation with a fast ventricular rate. In these circumstances an infusion of Digoxin 0.25 mg IV over 15 minutes is repeated to a maximum of 1.0–1.5 mg (assuming normal renal function), until the ventricular rate falls to <80/min. Although digoxin is well absorbed by the oral route, the normal function of the gastrointestinal tract is unreliable in the presence of a low cardiac output. Ectopic activity and digoxin induced arrhythmias can be minimised by maintaining the serum potassium >4.0 mmol/l with IV supplements. Other atrial or junctional arrhythmias are best treated DC countershock as this has less cardiodepressant action when compared with other antiarrhythmic drugs.

8. *Other measures*

Historical methods of controlling 'preload' using venesection or rotating tourniquets are seldom used today.

ADULT RESPIRATORY DISTRESS SYNDROME (SHOCK LUNG)

Adult respiratory distress syndrome (ARDS) or 'shock lung' is an increasingly recognised condition with an overall mortality of 40–60%. Acute respiratory failure in association with 'non-cardiac pulmonary oedema' can be caused by a variety of conditions (see p. 91), but the functional consequences of the pulmonary insult are similar.

Features of ARDS

1. Progressive arterial hypoxaemia
2. Reduced lung compliance and functional residual capacity
3. Increased dead space: tidal volume ratio
4. Increased work of breathing
5. Increased shunt fraction
6. Elevated PA pressure and PVR.

Pathophysiology

1. *Pulmonary artery occlusion*

Occlusion of branch or microscopic pulmonary arteries can be demonstrated in 50% of patients with ARDS, and is particulary common in association with trauma, burns and severe pulmonary infection. Whether occlusion represents in

situ thrombosis or pulmonary embolism is unclear.
Thrombocytopaenia occurs in 60% of patients and evidence
of disseminated intravascular coagulation (elevated FDPs)
may be present.

2. *Alveolar-capillary membrane disruption*
Intravascular injury, possibly related to local release of
vasoactive mediators (e.g. histamine, serotonin, thromboxane
A_2, PGF_2, and leukotrienes LTC_4 and $LTDD_4$), results in
leakage of protein and blood across the alveolar-capillary
membrane into the alveolar air spaces and the interstitium.
Furthermore, loss of colloid osmotic pressure leads to
alveolar flooding, inadequate ventilation, V/Q mismatch and
an increase in right to left shunting.

3. *Pulmonary fibrosis*
Within a few hours intra-alveolar protein coagulates and
there is necrosis of Type I pneumocytes (alveolar lining
cells), hyaline membrane deposition, and hyperplasia of Type
II pneumocytes (surfactant producing cells). Fibroblast
activation results in fibrosis (some of which may be
reversible) within seven days.

4. *Other factors*
In certain circumstances (e.g. cardiopulmonary bypass or
haemodialysis), further damage is caused by complement
(C_{5a}) activation. A high FIO_2 and free O_2 radicals (.OH,
O_2^-, H_2O_2) may compound the toxicity of certain agents
including paraquat and nitrofurantoin.

Clinical features

Following the initial insult (e.g. trauma, burns), there is a latent period
of approximately 24 hours during which time the patient may exhibit
hyperventilation, respiratory alkalosis and arterial hypoxaemia of variable
severity. The cause of the hyperventilation is not clear; it persists despite
the correction of hypoxaemia, and may represent reflex phenomenon as a
result of a reduction in lung compliance. Subsequently, the development
of pulmonary oedema and pulmonary arterial hypertension is associated
with progressive hypoxia, hypercarbia and death in some cases despite all
attempts to support the patient. Unlike the patient with pulmonary
oedema with an elevated PACWP, the cardiac output is maintained and
the patient appears warm and well perfused. Sepsis may be an important
accompaniment of ARDS late in the course of the illness.

Investigations

1. *Chest radiograph*
The chest radiograph remains normal for the first 24 hours,
but then undergoes a characteristic series of changes (Table

Table 5.4 Radiological features of adult respiratory distress syndrome

Stage	Radiology	Time
I	Normal chest radiograph	0–24 h
II	Interstitial and alveolar oedema	24–36 h
III	No change	36–72 h
IV	Improvement, resolution or death	72 h–6 weeks

5.4). In contrast to pulmonary oedema associated with an elevated PACWP, upper lobe blood diversion, cardiac enlargement and pleural effusions are not features of ARDS. A 35% increase in extravascular lung water can occur without any apparent abnormality on the chest radiograph.

2. *Arterial blood gases*
   Arterial hypoxaemia is more marked than in pulmonary oedema related to cardiac disease. Impaired diffusion does not contribute to the hypoxia, but the shunt fraction may approach 30% as a result of V/Q mismatch. Hypercarbia and metabolic acidosis are seen terminally.

Management

Prognosis in ARDS may be improved with intensive monitoring, strict control of fluid balance and nutrition, appropriate antibiotics, early mechanical ventilation and correction (if possible) of hypoxaemia. All patients should be monitored in an ICU, and in those requiring assisted ventilation, an indwelling arterial catheter and a thermodilution Swan-Ganz catheter to monitor PA pressure, PACWP and cardiac output are advantageous (see Ch. 20). This flow-directed catheter can also be used to perform selective balloon occlusion pulmonary arteriography using portable fluoroscopy at the bedside.

1. *Mechanical ventilation*
   An attempt is made to maintain the PaO_2 between 8 and 10 kPa (60–75 mmHg) on the lowest FIO_2 possible. A tidal volume of 15 ml/kg is appropriate, with a respiratory rate to maintain the $PaCO_2$ within the normal range (approximately 5 kPa, 35–40 mmHg). The addition of a positive end expiratory pressure (PEEP) valve on the expiratory limb of the ventilator usually allows a reduction in FIO_2 without a concomitant fall in PaO_2. PEEP increases the functional residual capacity (FRC), inflates collapsed and flooded air spaces, and improves V/Q mismatch. Venous return and cardiac output are reduced by PEEP, and the PVR may be increased. Radiological clearing following the addition of PEEP may precede improvement in blood gas status. Pulmonary barotrauma (pneumothorax, pneumomediastinum and surgical emphysema) is a major complication of PEEP.

Extracorporeal membrane oxygenation does not improve the prognosis in patients with severe ARDS, and high frequency ventilation (>3 Hz) cannot be recommended for adults, except in specialist units.

2. *Fluid management*

Resuscitation has been implicated as a factor in the development of ARDS. Frequently, excessive amounts of crystalloid are administered in an uncontrolled manner during resuscitation. When the patient is stable (following the initial insult), fluid replacement should be strictly controlled by means of the PACWP. Minimal fluids are given to maintain an adequate urine output (30 ml/h),with additional diuretics if necessary. Controversy exists as to whether crystalloid or colloid replacement is appropriate, but most authorities favour crystalloid replacement. All blood should be passed through a 20 micron micropore filter particularly when large transfusions are necessary (e.g. following trauma).

3. *Cardiac function*

Approximately 25% of patients with ARDS are found to have unsuspected left ventricular disease. Although PEEP has been shown to impair LV diastolic function, a direct effect on systolic function is less certain. Despite a reduction in venous return leading to a fall in cardiac output, little change in systemic blood pressure is seen on moderate levels of PEEP (10 cm H_2O), due to an increase in systemic vascular resistance secondary to a reflex sympathetic response. During conventional levels of PEEP (<20 cm H_2O), vagally mediated effects on venous return are unimportant. However, alpha adrenergic blockade exaggerates the reduction in venous return caused by PEEP.

4. *Corticosteroids*

The experimental observation that C_5 activation can be prevented by high doses of steroids may be one of the mechanisms by which corticosteroids reduce alveolar-capillary leakage (particularly in cases of sepsis). If steroids are used at all they should be given early as Methylprednisolone 30 mg/kg IV as a bolus which can be repeated once after 12 hours if necessary.

5. *Antibiotics*

Respiratory infection is a major cause of death in the patient with ARDS. Within three days of arriving in an ICU, 75% of patients will have bacterial colonisation of the upper airway, and as a result of impaired host defence mechanisms 20–30% will develop severe lower respiratory infections frequently due to gram negative bacilli. Many of these infections are endogenous (from the gastrointestinal tract) and are spread from patient to patient within the ICU by means of staff contact or shared equipment (e.g. ventilators).

Frequent sputum cultures are mandatory although they are often unhelpful because of a mixed growth of multiple organisms. Uncontaminated specimens from the lower respiratory tract can be obtained using transtracheal aspiration, fibreoptic bronchoscopy and brush biopsy, or transbronchial biopsy. All material should be examined for pyogenic organisms (including anaerobes), fungi and viral inclusions. Legionella may be identified directly by fluorescence, or by a serum complement fixation test. In cases of occult infection a [67]Gallium or Indium white cell scan may be helpful. The indiscriminate use of broad spectrum antibiotics encourages growth of resistant organisms and fungi; however, the rapid identificatiion of the pathogen is not always possible and not infrequently 'blind' treatment has to be instituted because of deterioration in the condition of the patient.

6. *Nutrition*

Maintaining adequate nutritional status is an important part of the management of the patient with ARDS. A low serum albumen and elevated blood urea may compound leakage of the alveolar-capillary membrane. The bowel is the preferred route for the administration of calories, but if gastrointestinal absorption is impaired parenteral nutrition will be required. Intravenous vitamin and trace element supplements are given to all patients who require supplement feeding for more than one week.

7. *Other measures*

Surface cooling (32–35°C) is indicated in the patient with a high fever (>39°C) in an attempt to reduce oxygen consumption and cardiac output. A prophylactic H_2 receptor antagonist (Cimetidine, Ranitidine) or regular antacids (Aluminium hydroxide) should be given to all patients with ARDS as there is a 30% incidence of gastrointestinal haemorrhage in this group of patients. Most authorities advocate low dose subcutaneous heparin (5000 units three times daily), but full anticoagulation is controversial and the role (if any) of thrombolytic agents is unclear. When disseminated intravascular coagulation complicates ARDS, platelet transfusions may be required to correct severe thrombocytopaenia.

Outcome

In the patient who has an extensive pulmonary infiltrate, a shunt fraction of >30% and a low PaO_2 despite an FIO_2 of 0.5–1.0 and PEEP, the mortality exceeds 90%. Death is usually preceded by an increasing

$PaCO_2$. In moderate ARDS, the chest radiograph shows some areas to be spared and adequate oxygenation can usually be maintained by mechanical ventilation using an FIO_2 of 0.5–0.8 without the addition of PEEP. The mortality in this group is approximately 50%. Most patients survive more minor episodes of ARDS in which blood gas abnormalities can be corrected wth supplemental oxygen without assisted ventilation.

6. MYOCARDIAL DISEASE

The cardiomyopathies are a group of conditions in which the primary abnormality affects the myocardium. In the majority of cases the aetiology is unclear — hence Goodwin's term 'heart muscle disease of unknown cause'. In a few patients myocardial dysfunction is a manifestation of a systemic disease (e.g. sarcoid), or is related to a drug or toxin (e.g. alcohol, adriamycin). It is inappropriate to use the term ischaemic cardiomyopathy for patients with left ventricular dysfunction secondary to coronary artery disease as the cause of the abnormality is known.

A functional classification is helpful to the understanding of the cardiomyopathies, although it is clear that these categories are not mutually exclusive because a patient may pass from one functional type of cardiomyopathy to another during the course of his illness (e.g. hypertrophic → dilated).

Functional classification of the cardiomyopathies:

1. *Hypertrophic*
   Severe ventricular hypertrophy that may be localised. Abnormalities of diastolic function. Dynamic outflow gradient.
2. *Dilated* (*congestive*)
   Dilated heart. Little hypertrophy. Impaired systolic function.
3. *Restrictive/obliterative*
   Abnormal ventricular filling. Moderate hypertrophy. Frequently associated with a systemic disorder (e.g. amyloid). Endocardial involvement may predominate (e.g. eosinophilic heart disease).

HYPERTROPHIC CARDIOMYOPATHY

Aetiology

The cause of hypertrophic cardiomyopathy is unknown but there are a number of aetiological factors that may be important:

1. *Inheritance*
   In a proportion of cases there is a genetic predisposition; in

some patients autosomal dominant inheritance has been documented and in others HLA linkage is seen.

2. *Catecholamines*

   Increased sensitivity or excess production of catecholamines has been implicated in hypertrophic cardiomyopathy. The association of hypertrophic cardiomyopathy with systemic hypertension, phaeochromocytoma, neurofibromatosis, lentiginosis and the occasional finding of hypertrophic cardiomyopathy in patients with hyperthyroidism and diabetes mellitus lends support to this concept. Furthermore, the response of hypertrophic cardiomyopathy to beta blocking drugs and the exacerbation by adrenergic agonists suggests that catecholamines are in some way involved in the condition.

3. *Ventricular structure and geometry*

   The abnormal (catenoid) shape of the ventricle in patients with hypertrophic cardiomyopathy favours isometric contraction which may bring about changes in ventricular structure (e.g. fibre disarray); other workers have emphasized the importance of abnormal ventricular activation as a cause of asynchronous contraction. Finally, an abnormal cardiac 'skeleton' as a result of a disorder of collagen synthesis has been postulated.

Pathology

Included in the term hypertrophic cardiomyopathy are a heterogeneous group of patients with ventricular hypertrophy. No single finding is specific or pathognomonic of hypertrophic cardiomyopathy but the following features may be found in a typical case:

1. *Ventricular hypertrophy*

   Asymmetric septal hypertrophy occurs in at least 90% of cases. Localised hypertrophy (e.g. apical) has also been described.

2. *Small ventricular cavity*

   Prominent papillary muscles encroach on the ventricular cavity which is small, slit-like and is obliterated in systole.

3. *Myocardial fibre disarray*

   Patchy disorganisation of myocardial fibres (whorls) is seen in 90% of patients and electron microscopy shows disarray of the myofibrils and myofilaments. Although these changes predominate in the ventricular septum they also occur elsewhere in the ventricle; furthermore, they are not diagnostic as they appear in some types of congenital heart disease and occasionally in normal subjects.

4. *Mural endocardial plaque*

   Endocardial thickening at the point of apposition of the

anterior leaflet of the mitral valve on the interventricular septum is seen in 75% of patients, particularly those with a severe out-flow tract gradient and systolic anterior movement (SAM) of the mitral valve on the echocardiogram (see p. 111).

5. *Abnormal mitral valve*
Thickening of the anterior (and less frequently) the posterior mitral leaflet where it impinges on the interventricular septum (as above).

6. *Atrial dilatation*
Increased ventricular stiffness and reduced compliance result in an increase in atrial pressure and atrial dilatation.

7. *Abnormal coronary arteries*
Increase in the number and size of the epicardial coronary arteries, together with hypertrophy of the intima and media is seen in 50% of patients with hypertrophic cardiomyopathy.

Pathophysiology (systolic vs diastolic abnormalities)

Emphasis in the early literature centred around the characteristic abnormalities of systolic function and the outflow tract gradient. It is now clear that the primary abnormality is diastolic, with impaired ventricular filling as a consequence of massive ventricular hypertrophy. If an outflow gradient is present at all it is dynamic and load dependent. Rather than left ventricular ejection being impeded, ventricular emptying is rapid and most of the antegrade flow precedes the development of an outflow tract gradient. The gradient is however responsible for a number of the clinical findings in hypertrophic cardiomyopathy; these include the characteristic nature of the arterial pulse, the late systolic murmur and systolic anterior movement of the mitral valve demonstrated by echocardiography.

Clinical history

1. *Asymptomatic*
More than 50% of patients with hypertrophic cardiomyopathy have no functional limitations and 20% are asymptomatic. One of the major difficulties with the management of these patients is that sudden death (see p. 256) may be the initial manifestation of the disease. Asymptomatic patients may come to medical attention because of an abnormal routine ECG or because of a positive family history. Elderly patients are often asymptomatic and in this sub-group the diagnosis may be an incidental finding at post mortem.

2. *Palpitations*
Episodes of sustained supraventricular or ventricular arrhythmias cause palpitations and may be provoked by

exertion or emotion. Arrhythmias are poorly tolerated because of the reduction in ventricular compliance and the important contribution of atrial transport.

3. *Breathlessness*
Elevation in the left ventricular end diastolic pressure and pulmonary venous hypertension cause progressive breathlessness. The onset of atrial fibrillation may provoke sudden dyspnoea.

4. *Chest pain*
Chest pain indistinguishable from angina pectoris is a common symptom in patients with hypertrophic cardiomyopathy. Possible mechanisms include altered coronary filling secondary to abnormal diastolic function, severe ventricular hypertrophy increasing myocardial oxygen requirements and concomitant coronary artery disease (either small vessel disease or atherosclerosis). Atypical chest pain may also occur.

5. *Loss of consciousness*
Dizziness or sudden loss of consciousness is usually related to episodes of tachyarrhythmia or ventricular standstill (rare). Severe outflow obstruction as a cause of syncope is probably overrated.

6. *Sudden death (see Ch. 16)*
Sudden death is a major cause of mortality in patients with hypertrophic cardiomyopathy. It appears to be related to ventricular fibrillation and is more common in athletes, young patients with a family history of sudden death, those with severe hypertrophy and patients with a malignant arrhythmia on a Holter monitor or provoked by exercise testing.

7. *Other symptoms*
A small minority of patients have symptoms related to an arterial embolism or infective endocarditis (see Ch. 11).

Physical examination

1. *General appearance*
Unless the cardiomyopathy is associated with one of the rare conditions in which there are abnormal physical characteristics (e.g. lentiginosis, neurofibromatosis etc.), the general appearance of the patient with hypertrophic cardiomyopathy is unremarkable. The incidence of the condition is bimodal with respect to age, 70% of patients being young adults and the remainder aged 60 years or more. Females and males are affected equally, but females tend to be younger and to have more severe disease.

2. *Venous pressure*
Typically the venous pressure is not raised, but there may be

a prominent 'a' wave reflecting the reduced ventricular compliance.

3. *Arterial pulse*

A normal volume pulse is characterised by a sharp upstroke which has a 'jerky' quality due to the sudden reduction in force of contraction in mid-systole coincident with the peak outflow gradient; a secondary rise (tidal wave) follows shortly thereafter resulting in a bisferiens pulse. A reduction in pulse pressure may be appreciated in the sinus beat following an ectopic (see post extrasystolic potentiation below). 20% of patients have systemic hypertension.

4. *Precordial impulses*

A sustained apex beat with a double impulse can be palpated and not infrequently a presystolic 'a' wave from atrial contraction can be appreciated as well. A systolic thrill may be present in patients with an outflow gradient.

5. *Heart sounds and murmurs*

In the absence of an outflow gradient auscultation of the heart may be normal. If there is a gradient the first sound is normal and the second sound is normal or A2 may be delayed due to severe left ventricular hypertrophy or LBBB. A fourth heart sound is common, as is a third sound, but there is no systolic ejection click. A variable late systolic murmur can be heard at the apex and there may be an ejection murmur at the lower left sternal edge. These murmurs are probably caused by mitral regurgitation and/or turbulence across the outflow tract. Murmurs at the base of the heart are uncommon. Manoeuvres that alter systemic arterial resistance (see Table 6.1) affect the intensity of the murmurs.

Table 6.1 Manoeuvres affecting the intensity of murmurs in patients with hypertrophic cardiomyopathy

Increase murmur
    Valsalva manoeuvre (straining phase)
    Standing
    Dynamic exercise
    Tachycardia
    Hypovolaemia
    Drugs (digoxin, amyl nitrite)
    Post extrasystolic potentiation

Decrease murmur
    Valsalva manoeuvre (overshoot phase)
    Mueller manoeuvre
    Squatting
    Isometric exercise
    Drugs (beta blockers, alpha agonists)

NB: Manoeuvres that tend to increase the intensity of the murmur increase the outflow gradient and vice versa

Investigations

1. *Blood tests*
   Routine blood tests are unhelpful in the diagnosis of hypertrophic cardiomyopathy. Plasma and urine levels of noradrenaline may be increased, but these changes are inconsistent and depend in part on the type of assay used.

2. *Electrocardiogram and Holter monitoring*
   Less than 10% of patients with hypertrophic cardiomyopathy have a normal ECG. Characteristic changes include repolarisation abnormalities with deep symmetrical T wave inversion and pathological Q waves particularly in the inferior or anterolateral leads are seen in up to 50% of patients. ECG features of left ventricular hypertrophy are the rule. Poor anterior R wave progression and Q waves occur secondary to septal hypertrophy, fibrosis or abnormal septal activation and do not necessarily imply myocardial ischaemia. Associated conduction abnormalities include left axis deviation, LBBB and pre-excitation (short PR interval) with or without a delta wave. Bradyarrhythmias and high grade atrioventricular block are rare. Most patients remain in sinus rhythm, but atrial fibrillation occurs in 5–10% of patients late in the course of their disease. Abnormalities of the P wave (biphasic P wave in V_1) reflect the elevation of left atrial pressure. Holter monitor recording demonstrates ventricular arrhythmias in 50–75% of patients, and malignant arrhythmias (e.g. ventricular tachycardia) occur in 25% of patients.

3. *Chest radiograph*
   50% of patients have a normal chest radiograph and even in the presence of severe ventricular hypertrophy the heart size may be normal. Left atrial dilatation may cause elevation of the left main bronchus resulting in a cardiac contour indistinguishable from mitral valve disease. An absence of aortic valve calcification and post-stenotic dilatation is useful in excluding aortic valve disease as the cause of the outflow gradient. Mitral annulus calcification is commonly associated with hypertrophic cardiomyopathy in elderly patients. Late in the course of the disease the heart enlarges and there may be evidence of an elevated left atrial pressure (interstitial oedema etc.).

4. *Echocardiography*
   Echocardiography is a unique method for the assessment of the patient with hypertrophic cardiomyopathy. Not only can the technique be used as a screening test or to follow individual patients in the long term, but it has also given considerable insight into the mechanisms involved in the

disease, particularly the abnormalities of diastolic function. A number of features of hypertrophic cardiomyopathy have been described on the M-mode echocardiogram (see Table 6.2); all have been described in other conditions, and none are specific for hypertrophic cardiomyopathy. Asymmetric septal hypertrophy (ASH) was initially said to be pathognomonic of hypertrophic cardiomyopathy, but it is now realised that ASH may occur in normal infants, athletes (e.g. weight lifters), in association with pulmonary hypertension and following inferior infarction. The degree of SAM relates to the severity of the outflow tract gradient. There is much overlap between the echocardiographic findings in hypertrophic cardiomyopathy and other types of secondary ventricular hypertrophy (e.g. in systemic hypertension). Diagnostic sensitivity and specificity is increased by documenting a number of the features listed and little emphasis should be placed on finding borderline ASH in isolation. M-mode echocardiography should always be combined with the cross-sectional technique as this allows the angulation of the septum to be accurately delineated. Increased echodensity and other abnormalities of echo texture also occur in other forms of ventricular hypertrophy and are therefore non-specific. Left ventricular thrombus and infective endocarditis, both well recognised complications of hypertrophic cardiomyopathy, may be confirmed by echocardiography.

5. *Radionuclide scanning*

Increase in left ventricular mass and the presence of asymmetric septal hypertrophy can be demonstrated by ^{201}Tl scintigraphy. In patients with chest pain in whom hypertrophic cardiomyopathy is a possible diagnosis the presence of a ^{201}Tl defect either at rest or on exercise is an unreliable method of diagnosing coronary artery disease because abnormal thallium scans have been described in patients with hypertrophic cardiomyopathy and normal coronary arteries. A reduction in ventricular cavity size

---

Table 6.2 Echocardiographic features of hypertrophic cardiomyopathy

 1. Septal hypertrophy
 2. Increased septal: posterior wall ratio (>1.3:1) (asymmetric septal hypertrophy — ASH)
 3. Systolic anterior movement of the mitral valve (SAM)
 4. Mid-systolic closure of the aortic valve
 5. Septal hypokinesis or akinesis
 6. Reduced LV end diastolic dimension
 7. Reduced septal-mitral valve separation
 8. Reduced mitral EF slope
 9. Prolonged and/or incoordinate ventricular relaxation
10. Increased left atrial dimension

together with the abnormalities gated of diastolic function can be appreciated using equilibrium blood pool scanning (MUGA) with ^{99m}Tc labelled autologous red cells. Echocardiography is superior to nuclear techniques in the follow-up of patients with hypertrophic cardiomyopathy.

6. *Exercise testing*

Arrhythmias may also be provoked by treadmill exercise testing but 24 hour ECG monitoring is a more sensitive technique in this respect. Of interest is the observation that the repolarisation changes noted on the resting ECG may normalise on exercise or following a small dose of a beta blocking drug, lending further support to the role of catecholamines in this condition.

7. *Haemodynamics*

Invasive investigation allows quantitation of the outflow gradient and can exclude additional valvular disease. Cardiac catheterisation is carried out using standard techniques (see Ch. 20) and great care should be taken to avoid spurious pressure readings being caused by the catheter becoming entrapped amongst the trabeculae or the mitral subvalve apparatus. A catheter-tipped Millar manometer is ideally suited for the purpose. A labile pressure gradient (if present) is likely to be detected in the body of the ventricle and a number of manoeuvres have been used to provoke or increase the gradient (Table 6.1) which in severe cases may be as high as 200 mmHg. If there is a significant gradient (>20 mmHg), the arterial pressure trace exhibits a 'spike and dome' pattern with a mid systolic dip and late systolic pressure rise. Decrease in ventricular compliance causes an increase in left and right atrial 'a' waves and a mild gradient may be detected across the right ventricular outflow tract secondary to septal hypertrophy. Cardiac output is maintained within the normal range until late in the disease.

Post extrasystolic potentiation is useful in determining the level of left ventricular outflow obstruction. In hypertrophic cardiomyopathy the pulse pressure is narrower in the post-ectopic beat than in the preceding sinus beat, whereas in normal subjects and in patients with other types of outflow obstruction the reverse is the case.

8. *Cineangiography*

A long axial view (see Ch. 20) permits the ventricular septum to be profiled, and the abnormal position of the mitral valve can be clearly visualised; furthermore, angled views allow differentiation between hypertrophic cardiomyopathy and other forms of discrete subaortic stenosis. Ventricular hypertrophy may be extreme resulting in a narrow slit-like cavity which is obliterated in mid-systole by the hypertrophied papillary muscles which causes contrast to be trapped in the apex of the ventricle. If mitral regurgitation is present it is seldom severe. Aortography should be carried out in all patients to exclude additional aortic regurgitation. Coronary arteriography usually reveals large smooth epicardial coronary arteries which may show discrete areas of smooth circumscribed indentation from muscle bridging. Concomitant organic coronary artery disease may also occur.

9. *Endomyocardial biopsy*

Typical histological features of hypertrophic cardiomyopathy include myocardial cell hypertrophy and fibre disarray. Foci of abnormal cells may be seen in biopsies of either ventricle (see Ch. 20 for details of the technique). However, endomyocardial biopsy is not necessary for an accurate diagnosis to be made in most cases.

Differential diagnosis

1. *Aortic valve stenosis*
2. *Subaortic stenosis*
   Discrete   } −see Chapter 9
   Tunnel
3. Supravalvar stenosis
4. Coronary artery disease   −see Chapter 1

Management

Medical

Agents causing arterial vasodilatation and a reduction in systemic vascular resistance (e.g. nitrates) should be avoided as they tend to exacerbate the outflow gradient. Similarly, inotropic agents are contraindicated in patients with hypertrophic cardiomyopathy unless the patient has end-stage myopathy by which time the nature of the ventricular disease is more of the dilated type. Digoxin is only used in certain specific circumstances (see p. 114). Patients with hypertrophic cardiomyopathy have non-compliant ventricles that require a high filling pressure, therefore diuretics should be used with caution. Patients who are asymptomatic with only mild abnormalities on the ECG or echocardiogram require no specific treatment, but should be followed up by echocardiography and Holter monitoring on a regular basis.

The following agents have a role in the treatment of hypertrophic cardiomyopathy:

1. *Beta receptor blockers*

Up to 70% of patients respond favourably to beta blockade, particularly those whose predominant symptom is chest pain rather than breathlessness. Beta blockers reduce myocardial contractility (peak dp/dt), lower myocardial oxygen requirements, increase left ventricular compliance and reduce the chronotropic response to exercise. Non-selective beta blockers (e.g Propranolol) limit the magnitude of the outflow gradient provoked by exertion and are preferable to the 'cardioselective' preparations in this respect. Beta blockers do not significantly reduce the resting gradient. An initial dose of Propranolol LA 160 mg once daily may be adequate, but some patients require much larger doses for symptomatic relief.

2. *Calcium channel blockers*
   Both verapamil and nifedipine have been used in patients with hypertrophic cardiomyopathy. Not only are they effective in treating chest pain, but there is experimental evidence showing that they may improve diastolic function. Small initial doses (e.g. verapamil 40 mg three times daily or nifedipine 10 mg three times daily) should be increased to the maximum tolerated dose. Side effects include fluid retention, facial flushing and systemic hypotension. Pre-existing conduction disorders are a relative contraindication to the use of calcium channel blockers. Although the combination of beta blocking drugs and calcium channel blockers is not generally recommended they have been successfully used in these patients. It is advisable to start this combination in hospital.

3. *Digoxin*
   Reduced ventricular compliance means that atrial arrhythmias and the associated loss of atrial transport are poorly tolerated in patients with hypertrophic cardiomyopathy. If DC countershock is ineffective in restoring sinus rhythm, then digoxin should be started in an attempt to control the ventricular rate. Occasional patients require the addition of small doses of a beta blocker (e.g. Propranolol 10 or 20 mg twice daily) for adequate rate control. At this stage digoxin can be used with little risk because atrial fibrillation occurs late in the natural history of hypertrophic cardiomyopathy at which time there is little or no outflow gradient.

4. *Amiodarone*
   Malignant ventricular arrhythmias may respond to therapy with amiodarone, and there is some evidence to suggest that the overall prognosis may be improved by this drug. A standard loading dose of amiodarone 600 mg once daily is given for two weeks followed by the minimum maintenance dose necessary to control the arrhythmia on an ECG tape (usually 200 mg once daily). Pre-existing conduction defects are a contraindication to amiodarone. Numerous side-effects have been reported with amiodarone and are listed in Chapter 16.

5. *Other antiarrhythmic drugs*
   Disopyramide, mexilitene and quinidine are rarely successful in controlling the arrhythmias associated with hypertrophic cardiomyopathy.
6. *Anticoagulants*
   With the onset of atrial fibrillation intravenous heparin should be commenced, initially using a continuous infusion of heparin 40 000 units/24 h, with the dose subsequently adjusted according to the KCT or thrombin time. If DC cardioversion is unsuccessful then warfarin is administered indefinitely according to the standard protocol.
7. *Endocarditis prophylaxis*
   Infective endocarditis affecting the mitral valve, aortic valve or mural endocardial plaque occurs in up to 10% of patients. Appropriate prophylactic antibiotics should be given for dental procedures and other potentially septic hazards (Ch. 11).

Surgery

1. *Septal myotomy and myectomy*
   Operative intervention is reserved for patients in whom medical treatment has failed. An incision into the ventricular septum (myotomy) or partial resection of the septum (myectomy) will correct mitral regurgitation and relieve the outflow gradient in most patients. Either a transaortic or direct left ventricular approach may be used, with an operative mortality of 5–10%.
2. *Mitral valve replacement*
   Occasional reports of mitral valve replacement (and removal of the hypertrophied papillary muscles) in patients with severe hypertrophic cardiomyopathy indicate that valve replacement leads to an increase in left ventricular cavity size and an improvement in diastolic compliance.

Natural history (can it be modified?)

Annual mortality in patients with hypertrophic cardiomyopathy is 4–6%. Sudden death is a major cause of mortality and appears to be more common in young patients (who may have been asymptomatic), those with a family history of sudden death and patients who experience syncopal episodes. Of interest is the rare occurrence of sudden death in patients with severe symptoms of chest pain and breathlessness. Beta blocking drugs do not influence the incidence of sudden death, but there is some evidence to suggest that amiodarone not only reduces the incidence of ventricular arrhythmias but also lowers the incidence of sudden death.

In the 'typical' patient with hypertrophic cardiomyopathy, symptoms begin in the third decade and progress slowly throughout adult life.

Sudden death may occur at any time, but atrial fibrillation is seen in old age. Symptoms from pulmonary oedema and fluid retention as a consequence of a dilated heart are uncommon. Pregnancy is well tolerated (see Ch. 18).

DILATED CARDIOMYOPATHY

Dilated (or congestive) cardiomyopathy is characterised by global impairment of systolic function and represents the final common pathway of many forms of ventricular disease. It is an uncommon condition with an incidence of 10 per 100 000 of the population. Occasionally patients with either hypertrophic or restrictive cardiomyopathy (e.g. amyloid) develop pathophysiology typical of dilated cardiomyopathy.

Aetiology

By definition, the cause of dilated cardiomyopathy is unknown (or idiopathic) and it is therefore a diagnosis of exclusion. Numerous causes of myocardial disease result in a clinical and functional picture indistinguishable from idiopathic dilated cardiomyopathy (Table 6.3) and the term 'dilated cardiomyopathy' is often used to refer to these patients. To avoid the semantics of nomenclature it is preferable to use a term like 'alcoholic heart muscles disease' when the aetiology of the condition can be identified. The relationship between viral myocarditis and post-viral dilated cardiomyopathy is discussed in Chapter 12.

Pathophysiology

Cavity dilatation affects all four cardiac chambers but is most marked in the left and right ventricles. If ventricular hypertrophy is present it is seldom impressive and is inadequate to compensate for the degree of cavity dilatation. Early in the natural history of the condition, cardiac output is maintained by an increase in heart rate which compensates for the reduction in stroke volume. Eventually end systolic volume increases

Table 6.3 Some causes of dilated (congestive) cardiomyopathy

1. Idiopathic dilated cardiomyopathy
2. Post viral
3. Systemic hypertension
4. Alcohol excess
5. Nutritional deficiency (e.g. thiamine)
6. Endocrine disorders (e.g. hyperthyroidism, diabetes mellitus)
7. Cardiotoxic drugs (e.g. adriamycin, cobalt)
8. Postpartum
9. Infiltration (e.g. amyloid, sarcoidosis)*

* Usually cause restrictive disease

with a concomitant increase in wall stress (Laplace), hence cardiac work and myocardial oxygen requirements increase.

Dilatation of the mitral and tricuspid annulus and malalignment of the papillary muscles causes mitral and/or tricuspid regurgitation. Usually it is clear that the primary abnormality is one of ventricular disease with secondary atrioventricular valve regurgitation; occasionally there may be doubt as to whether the valve dysfunction itself is the primary abnormality (see Ch. 8).

Global impairment of systolic function causes a reduction in ejection phase indices (ejection fraction, peak VCF etc.) and the reduction in forward flow may permit mural thrombus to accumulate within the cardiac chambers. Abnormalities of diastolic function are secondary to the systolic disorder.

Clinical history

Idiopathic dilated cardiomyopathy most commonly affects middle-aged men. Symptoms are insidious and relate to a low cardiac output and pulmonary venous hypertension as a consequence of a raised left ventricular end diastolic pressure (Table 6.4).

Physical findings

1. *General appearance*
   In long-standing disease the patient appears thin and emaciated. A low cardiac output causes cool extremities and peripheral cyanosis. Chronic elevation of the central venous pressure leads to ankle oedema, ascites and mild icterus.
2. *Venous pressure*
   Elevation of the venous pressure may be marked with prominence of the 'a' wave, a poor 'x' descent and a large systolic ('cv') wave. Ventricular premature beats may be identified as cannon waves in the jugular venous pulse.
3. *Arterial pulse*
   A rapid, small volume pulse is typical. Systemic blood pressure is often maintained by peripheral vasoconstriction and a rise in systemic vascular resistance. Severe disease may be accompanied by pulsus alternans.

Table 6.4 Symptoms in dilated cardiomyopathy

1. Breathlessness, orthopnoea, and nocturnal dyspnoea
2. Fatigue and lethargy
3. Anorexia and abdominal pain (gut and hepatic congestion)
4. Fluid retention
5. Prior history of a viral illness
6. Symptoms related to systemic embolism
7. Chest pain (pulmonary embolism)
8. Initial symptoms may be precipitated by a lower respiratory infection

4. *Precordial impulses*

Cardiac dilatation causes the apical impulse to be displaced laterally and a presystolic 'a' wave may be palpable. Little apical movement is usual and a dynamic apex beat suggests that mitral regurgitation is severe and myocardial dysfunction may be a secondary phenomenon. Left ventricular hypertrophy is rarely severe enough to cause a sustained apex beat.

5. *Heart sounds and murmurs*

S1 is normal. S2 is narrowly split with an accentuated pulmonary component if there is pulmonary hypertension. In severe left ventricular disease or LBBB left ventricular ejection is prolonged and S2 may be single or reversed. Elevation in left atrial pressure causes an audible S4 and an S3 (during rapid ventricular filling) is almost invariable. Sinus tachycardia shortens diastole and a single mid-diastolic sound is heard, the so-called summation gallop. Dilatation of the atrioventricular annulus results in a late systolic murmur which develops into a pansystolic murmur when the regurgitation increases in severity. A palpable thrill seldom occurs in dilated cardiomyopathy. Exercise exacerbates mitral regurgitation and the increased venous return associated with inspiration accentuates the murmur of tricuspid regurgitation.

6. *Systemic embolism*

Sudden abdominal or limb pain, or a cerebrovascular event may be indicative of a systemic embolism.

7. *Optic fundi*

Physical examination should include careful evaluation of the optic fundi for evidence of pre-existing systemic hypertension.

8. *No physical signs*

In early disease physical signs may be absent at rest but become apparent on exercise.

Investigations

1. *Blood tests*

Routine blood tests are usually unhelpful. Deranged hepatic function may reflect passive congestion and a 'hepatitic' picture with an elevated gamma glutamyl transpeptidase and a macrocytosis (elevated MCV) is compatible with alcohol excess. Cardiac enzymes are normal and a viral screen is usually negative.

2. *Electrocardiogram*

Most patients with dilated cardiomyopathy have an abnormal ECG but this is unhelpful in differentiating ischaemic from idiopathic heart muscle disease. Sinus tachycardia at rest is indicative of impaired left ventricular function. 25% of patients are in atrial fibrillation. Simple or complex ventricular arrhythmias are common and further reduce the cardiac output. Intermittent or sustained ventricular tachycardia occurs in 25% of patients on a routine 12 lead ECG and a further 15% have ventricular tachycardia on a Holter monitor or during a formal exercise test. A biphasic P wave reflects the elevated left atrial pressure. Mean frontal QRS axis is abnormal in 50% of patients and 10% have LBBB or an interventricular conduction defect. High grade atrioventricular block is rare. Poor anterior R wave progression or septal Q waves are due to abnormal septal depolarisation and are not necessarily indicative of ischaemic heart disease. Left ventricular hypertrophy on voltage criteria may be present. Non-specific repolarisation abnormalities (ST segment depression, T wave flattening or inversion) are common.

3. *Chest radiograph*
   Cardiac enlargement is more marked than in either hypertrophic or restrictive cardiomyopathy. Dilatation of both ventricles and atria often in association with a pericardial effusion contribute to the overall increase in radiographic heart size. The superior vena cava and azygos vein may be prominent and pleural effusions are common. Patients with dilated cardiomyopathy are at risk from pulmonary embolism or pulmonary infarction which may be apparent on the chest radiograph (see Ch. 14). Features of an elevated left atrial pressure (upper lobe blood diversion, interstitial and alveolar oedema) accompany severe disease (see Ch. 5).

4. *Echocardiography*
   M-mode and cross-sectional echocardiography demonstrate dilatation of all four cardiac chambers, particularly the left atrium and left ventricle. End systolic and end diastolic dimensions are increased and fractional shortening is reduced. Unlike ischaemic heart disease which affects segmental wall motion, left ventricular function is globally impaired in dilated cardiomyopathy. Left ventricular aneurysm is in the differential diagnosis of dilated cardiomyopathy and although a left ventricular aneurysm may be identified by ultrasound it cannot be excluded with certainty. If left ventricular hypertrophy is present it is mild. Mural thrombus may be apparent in any cardiac chamber but is most common in the left ventricle. Dilatation of the atrioventricular annulus may cause incomplete coaption of either the mitral or the tricuspid valve leaflets during ventricular systole. Organic valve disease can be excluded by echocardiography, but low forward flow may cause incomplete mitral or aortic opening

and premature closure. If a pericardial effusion is present it can be readily identified and quantitated.

5. *Radionuclide scanning*

Left ventricular ejection fraction can be estimated by gated blood pool scanning using ^{99m}Tc-pertechnetate (MUGA), and this technique is useful in differentiating global from segmental ventricular disease. Sensitivity is increased by means of an exercise study (see Ch. 20). Myocardial perfusion imaging with [201]Thallium cannot readily differentiate between ischaemic and idiopathic left ventricular disease.

6. *Haemodynamics*

Left ventricular end diastolic pressure and pulmonary artery capillary wedge pressure are elevated to a greater extent than than the right-sided pressures. Prominence of a systolic 'cv' wave in the atrial pressure trace is indicative of mitral or tricuspid regurgitation, but the actual value is more dependent on atrial size. Indices of systolic function are impaired and cardiac output and index are reduced. Careful evaluation of the outflow tract is mandatory because a small outflow tract gradient may be significant if the cardiac output is low.

7. *Cineangiography*

Left ventricular cineangiography reveals a dilated ventricle with global hypokinesia. Ejection fraction is reduced and end diastolic volume is increased. Mural thrombus may be apparent, usually along the inferior wall or in the apex of the left ventricle. Mild degrees of mitral regurgitation are common but estimation of the severity of the lesion may be difficult if the atrium is very large. Coronary arteriography is either normal, or shows mild disease insufficient to account for the degree of ventricular dysfunction.

8. *Endomyocardial biopsy*

Routine use of endomyocardial biopsy in patients with idiopathic dilated cardiomyopathy is controversial. Alcoholic heart muscle disease cannot be differentiated with certainty from idiopathic cardiomyopathy, and as these two groups of patients constitute the majority of patients who are investigated with dilated hearts, cardiac biopsy does not appear to be justifiable. In occasional patients a tissue diagnosis is very helpful, for example histological grading of cardiotoxicity due to adriamycin therapy is the only method of accurately estimating the degree of cardiac injury, thereby allowing the dose of the drug to be adjusted for an individual patient. Furthermore, histological evaluation of the myocardium is the only possible technique for differentiating dilated cardiomyopathy and myocarditis and even then there may be difficulty in distinguishing the two conditions by histology. Trials of corticosteroids or other immuno-suppressive agents cannot be recommended without a tissue diagnosis. The role of endomyocardial biopsy in the diagnosis and management of myocarditis is discussed in Chapter 12.

Differential diagnosis

1. *Ischaemic heart disease*
   Chest pain is the major symptom in the patient with coronary artery disease, whereas breathlessness is the main complaint in dilated cardiomyopathy. Episodes of 'silent' infarction in which chest pain is not a prominent feature occurs in the elderly and patients with diabetes mellitus. The segmental nature of ischaemic heart muscle disease may be apparent on cross-sectional echocardiography and can be confirmed with cineangiography and coronary arteriography. When multiple infarcts have occurred left ventricular function may resemble that seen in dilated cardiomyopathy.
2. *Myocarditis*
   See Chapter 12.

Management

General measures
It makes sense to restrict the activities of the patient if he is symptomatic, particularly when there has been a sudden deterioration in exercise tolerance. Activities should be tailored to meet individual limitations, and competitive sport or other forms of isometric exercise must be avoided. Data showing the beneficial effects of bedrest on prognosis are less certain and prolonged bedrest may have a detrimental psychological effect on the patient. Bedrest does however permit some control over dietary intake and may be the only method of ensuring complete abstinence from alcohol in the alcoholic patient. A no salt diet is unpalatable and can be circumvented by using larger doses of diuretics as necessary; a no-added salt diet (approximately 150 mg/24 h) is a reasonable compromise. Attention to the serum potassium (ie maintaining $K^+ > 4.0$ mmol/1) is important in those patients who are prone to arrhythmias.

Drugs
Whereas the management of dilated cardiomyopathy used to be dependent on digoxin and diuretics, recent progress in the understanding of cardiovascular pathophysiology has led to the widespread use of vasodilator therapy. Instead of stimulating the heart with inotropic agents thereby increasing myocardial oxygen consumption (MVO_2) or reducing

the intravascular volume with diuretics, the judicious use of combinations of venous and arterial vasodilators allows redistribution of the intravascular volume to optimise cardiac loading. In many centres vasodilators are the first-line of treatment for dilated cardiomyopathy and diuretics and/or inotropic agents are added later if necessary. Right heart catheterisation using a Swan-Ganz catheter (see Ch. 20) may be necessary for the selection of drugs and 'fine tuning' in a particular patient. However, clinical examination will usually confirm whether the problem is mainly pulmonary venous congestion and an elevation in 'preload' (when a venodilator will be required), or whether the primary abnormality is a low cardiac output and poor tissue perfusion (which is an indication for an arterial dilator).

1. *Arterial and venodilators* (see Ch. 7).

2. *Diuretics*
   Excessive doses of diuretics are frequently prescribed for patients with dilated cardiomyopathy. Over diuresis causes a reduction in 'preload', fall in cardiac output, postural dizziness, hyponatraemia, metabolic alkalosis, pre-renal azotaemia and hyperuricaemia. The most effective diuresis can be achieved using a combination of a loop diuretic (e.g. Frusemide) with an agent working on the distal nephron (e.g. thiazides, amiloride, triamterene). Frusemide 80 mg po once or twice daily + Moduretic or Dyazide one or two po daily is a useful combination. This also avoids the need for oral potassium supplements which may cause gastrointestinal upset. Excessive diuresis may be clinically apparent from a reduction in skin turgor, postural hypotension, cool peripheries, anorexia, nausea and vomiting.

3. *Digoxin*
   Use of digoxin in the patient in sinus rhythm is controversial. Digoxin has been shown to increase myocardial contractility (e.g. peak dp/dt), and to shift favourably the myocardial function curve. Cardiac output is increased and there is a direct action of digoxin on renal tubular function to inhibit sodium reabsorption. These effects may be short-lived and the beneficial actions must be weighed against the numerous side-effects of the drug (see Ch. 16). Digoxin is indicated for the patient with dilated cardiomyopathy and atrial fibrillation if DC countershock has failed.

4. *Other oral inotropes (amrinone, milrinone etc.)*
   A new group of inotropic agents which do not act via catecholamines, histamine receptors or Na^+-K^+ ATPase activity. Amrinone appears to improve myocardial contractility without increasing MVO_2. Serious side-effects including thrombocytopaenia and gastrointestinal intolerance limits the usefulness of amrinone, but the newer agent milrinone may be less toxic.

5. *Antiarrhythmic drugs*

Episodes of sustained tachycardia, or frequent atrial or ventricular premature beats can seriously reduce cardiac output. In the absence of a correctable cause (e.g. electrolyte disturbance) the administration of antiarrhythmic agents may be appropriate. These drugs should be used with caution as they all depress myocardial function to a variable degree. Details of individual drugs are given in Chapter 16.

6. *Anticoagulants*

Prophylaxis against deep venous thrombosis (Heparin 5000 units sc three times daily) is advisable for the patient when mobility is restricted. If left ventricular thrombus is visualised by echocardiography or cineangiography the patient should be fully anticoagulated with intravenous heparin followed by warfarin. Similarly, full anticoagulation is advisable for patients who have sustained a major arterial embolism.

7. *Oxygen*

Supplemental oxygen is only necessary if the PaO_2 is <8kPa (on air), or the SaO_2 is <90%. This is uncommon in uncomplicated dilated cardiomyopathy.

8. *Beta adrenergic blockers*

Over the last few years a number of groups have shown that small doses of beta blockers (e.g. Metoprolol 2.5–5 mg po twice daily) not only improve ventricular function in some patients with dilated cardiomyopathy but also prolong survival. Some rational basis for this controversial form of therapy is now available. The failing heart is subjected to increased concentrations of circulating catecholamines and in these circumstances myocardial beta receptors appear to loose their sensitivity and there is an additional reduction in receptor numbers. Administration of adrenergic agonists may actually be detrimental because they will exacerbate receptor 'down-regulation'. Administration of beta blockers has been shown to increase beta receptor density in man, providing a partial explanation for improved ventricular function documented in these patients. At present this treatment is experimental and cannot be recommended for routine use.

9. *Vitamins*

Not only does alcohol have a direct myocardial depressant action, but the nutritional deficiency (particularly thiamine deficiency) seen in many alcoholics may also be important in the pathogenesis of alcoholic heart muscle disease. During hospital admission high dose vitamins (e.g. Parentrovite IVHP, one pair of ampoules IV daily for three days) should be given, followed by oral vitamin supplements (e.g. Orovite two tablets daily) indefinitely. Rarely is the response to vitamins very impressive, which is in contrast to the improvement seen with vitamin supplements in other nutritional causes of heart muscle disease (e.g. Oriental beriberi).

Surgery

Exclusion of localised or segmental left ventricular disease (e.g. left ventricular aneurysm) is important as it can be treated by conventional cardiac surgery (i.e. aneurysm resection ± coronary artery bypass grafting). Occasional patients benefit from mitral valve replacement when the mitral regurgitation is thought to be a significant factor in the left ventricular dysfunction. The decision to perform mitral valve replacement should not be undertaken lightly because the mitral regurgitation may actually be assisting ventricular performance by unloading the ventricle.

Cardiac transplantation is now a therapeutic option for patients with idiopathic dilated cardiomyopathy. At Stanford University Medical Centre where more than 400 patients have now undergone cardiac transplantation, 40% had dilated cardiomyopathy. With the advent of cyclosporine, actuarial survival for all patients is now 82% at one year and 74% at two years after transplantation. Many other centres throughout the world are now achieving success rates approaching the Stanford experience.

Prognosis

Patients with ventricular arrhythmias, systemic embolism, cardiac enlargement of depressed contractility have a two year mortality of 50%, and an eight year mortality of 77%. Of the patients referred for transplantation, few are living after six months. Factors that adversely affect the prognosis include an LVEDP >20 mmHg, a cardiothoracic ratio >0.55 and a cardiac index <3.0 $1/min/m^2$. In most series spontaneous regression has been documented in approximately 5% of patients.

RESTRICTIVE CARDIOMYOPATHY

Restrictive cardiomyopathy is the least common of the cardiomyopathies and is typified by abnormal diastolic function as a result of reduced ventricular compliance. Depending on the aetiology of the restrictive process, varying degrees of atrioventricular valvar regurgitation, or conduction abnormalities may form part of the clinical picture. Clinical and haemodynamic similarities between restrictive cardiomyopathy and constrictive pericarditis may make differentiation of the two conditions difficult or impossible.

Aetiology

Although a number of infiltrative processes may give rise to a cardiomyopathy (Table 6.5), the cause of the restriction is unknown in most cases. By definition the term restrictive cardiomyopathy is limited to patients with primary myocardial disease and therefore excludes patients in whom ventricular hypertrophy and a reduced ventricular volume leads to impaired filling (e.g. aortic stenosis). Nor should the term be used in patients who have impaired systolic function and additional abnormalities of diastolic function (e.g. dilated cardiomyopathy).

Occasional patients do not fit neatly into any particular category of cardiomyopathy in which case a description of the clinical findings, haemodynamics and pathology is all that is possible.

Pathophysiology

As a consequence of reduced ventricular compliance (compliance = change in volume per unit change in pressure), elevated ventricular filling pressures are associated with normal (or near normal) systolic function. In contrast to hypertrophic cardiomyopathy, diastolic filling is limited but not prolonged. Depending on the aetiology of the restriction either left or right-sided disease may predominate.

Clinical history

Symptoms are attributable to the fixed cardiac output and the elevation in the central venous pressure.

1. Fatigue
2. Anorexia and weight loss
3. Fluid retention and abdominal distension
4. Chest pain (uncommon)
5. Symptoms related to a systemic disorder (e.g. amyloid, sarcoid, neoplasia)

Table 6.5 Causes of restrictive cardiomyopathy

1. Idiopathic restrictive cardiomyopathy
2. Amyloid
3. Sarcoidosis
4. Eosinophilic heart disease
5. Endomyocardial fibrosis
6. Neoplastic infiltration
7. Haemochromatosis and haemosiderosis
8. Glycogen storage diseases
9. Fabry's disease
10. Whipple's disease
11. Carcinoid
12. African cardiomyopathy (Becker's disease)

Physical findings

1. *General appearance*
   Wasting and emaciation may be striking. Lower limb oedema, ascites and hepatic enlargement occur in long-standing disease.

2. *Venous pressure*
   Increase in the venous pressure with deep 'x' and 'y' descents gives the characteristic 'M' or 'W' waveform, and the venous pressure *may* increase on inspiration (Kussmaul's sign), although this is less marked than in patients with pericardial constriction. Tricuspid regurgitation is accompanied by a prominent systolic ('cv') wave.

3. *Precordial impulses*
   Unlike pericardial constriction, the apex beat is usually palpable.

4. *Heart sounds and murmurs*
   S1 is normal and the pulmonary component of S2 may be accentuated. An early S3, coincident with the rapid filling wave of the apexcardiogram is typical of restrictive cardiomyopathy, and an S4 is frequently audible. A pansystolic murmur from mitral and/or tricuspid regurgitation can be heard in some forms of restrictive disease.

Investigations

1. *Blood tests*
   Abnormalities of liver function are seen in patients with hepatic congestion. Other helpful diagnostic pointers in the peripheral blood include hypercalcaemia in sarcoidosis, eosinophilia in some forms of eosinophilic cardiomyopathy, and elevated serum iron and transferrin in haemochromatosis.

2. *Electrocardiogram*
   Non-specific abnormalities of the electrocardiogram are common. Approximately 50% of patients are in atrial fibrillation which is poorly tolerated because of loss of atrial transport and abbreviated ventricular filling. In obliterative forms of cardiomyopathy (e.g. endomyocardial fibrosis) the reduction in stroke volume results in a compensatory tachycardia. Small voltage complexes, poor R wave progression and non-specific repolarisation abnormalities are often present. Sinoatrial block or atrioventricular conduction abnormalities may occur and are particularly common in sarcoidosis and cardiac amyloid.

3. *Chest radiograph*
   A normal cardiothoracic ratio helps to exclude other forms of ventricular disease (see p. 96, Table 5.3). In predominantly

right-sided disease the chest radiograph is unimpressive. showing a dilated superior vena cava and oligaemic lung fields. In left-sided disease the features of an elevated left atrial pressure are apparent (see Ch. 5). Pericardial calcification is occasionally seen.

4. *Echocardiography*

   Concentric left ventricular hypertrophy can be demonstrated by M-mode or cross-sectional echocardiography. Unlike hypertrophic cardiomyopathy cavity dimensions are normal and other echocardiographic features of hypertrophic cardiomyopathy (e.g. systolic anterior movement of the mitral valve) are absent. Systolic function is preserved except in late disease, but the abnormalities of diastolic function, particularly the sudden halting of ventricular filling in early diastole can be readily appreciated. Echocardiographic features of amyloid include increased myocardial echodensity (most marked in the interventricular septum), increased thickness of the interatrial septum and atrial free wall and small pericardial effusions. In eosinophilic heart disease apical cavity obliteration may be apparent in one or both ventricles. *NB*: The finding of left ventricular hypertrophy on the echocardiogram with small complexes on the ECG supports a diagnosis of restrictive cardiomyopathy rather than hypertrophic cardiomyopathy.

5. *Haemodynamics*

   Elevation of the mean right atrial pressure with deep 'x' and 'y' descents *may* show an increase in pressure on inspiration. Elevation in PACWP is more marked than that in the right atrium, and is accentuated by exercise. Prominent 'v' waves in either the right atrial or the PACWP trace indicates atrioventricular valve regurgitation due to the infiltration affecting the subvalve apparatus or less commonly the valves themselves. A 'dip and plateau' or 'square root sign' is present in the ventricular pressure trace, representing a deep early diastolic descent followed by a prolonged period of diastasis. Elevation in pulmonary arterial pressure is more marked than in patients with constrictive pericarditis and equalisation of the ventricular end diastolic pressures is uncommon in restrictive cardiomyopathy. Indices of systolic function are usually normal.

6. *Cineangiography*

   Ventricular volumes are normal but concentric hypertrophy may be marked. There is evidence of global ventricular disease with no regional wall motion abnormalities. Sudden halting of diastolic filling may be apparent but is probably best demonstrated by echocardiography. In obliterative forms of cardiomyopathy, the apical region of the ventricle appears 'cut off' by endocardial disease with overlying thrombus.

7. *Endomyocardial biopsy*

This technique is a simple and safe procedure that allows the cause of the cardiomyopathy to be determined with certainty in many patients. Biopsy of either the left or the right ventricle is undertaken at the time of cardiac catheterisation.

Differential diagnosis

Distinguishing features of restrictive cardiomyopathy, constrictive pericarditis and cardiac tamponade are discussed in Chapter 13.

Management

1. *Drugs*

Patients with restrictive cardiomyopathy tolerate drugs poorly. Excessive diuresis causes a reduction in intravascular volume which reduces cardiac output due to an inadequate preload. Similarly, venous and arterial dilators are rarely beneficial. A few reports indicate that ventricular compliance may be improved with calcium channel blockers (nifedipine, verapamil, diltiazem), and a cautious trial of one of these agents is worthwhile as the therapeutic options in this condition are limited. Corticosteroids and/or other immunosuppressive agents may be appropriate for patients with eosinophilic heart disease. Conduction abnormalities complicating sarcoidosis may regress with steroids in the occasional patient. Desferrioxamine and venesection may be beneficial in haemochromatosis.

2. *Pacing*

Symptomatic sinoatrial disease and high trade atrioventricular block (see Ch. 17) are indications for permanent endocardial pacing. A high output unit may be required because endocardial infiltration can increase the threshold necessary for capture.

3. *Surgery*

Resection of the thickened endocardium with or without atrioventricular valve replacement may be indicated in endomyocardial fibrosis or eosinophilic heart disease. If there is reasonable doubt as to whether a patient is suffering from restrictive cardiomyopathy or constrictive pericarditis, then exploratory thoracotomy should be undertaken. Cardiac transplantation is not appropriate for most patients with restrictive cardiomyopathy because the condition is likely to recur in the graft.

7. VASODILATOR THERAPY

PHYSIOLOGY OF THE FAILING HEART

Pharmacological manipulation of the loading conditions of the failing heart by vasodilator drugs is currently the primary method of treating the patient with impaired myocardial function complicating acute myocardial infarction or dilated cardiomyopathy. In the subgroup of patients in whom vasodilator therapy alone is ineffective then inotropic agents may be combined with vasodilators if optimum loading fails to provide adequate tissue perfusion.

Satisfactory myocardial metabolism is dependent on a balance between oxygen supply and demand (Table 7.1); the aim of vasodilator therapy is to reduce myocardial oxygen consumption (MVO_2) and hence cardiac work.

Many factors contribute to overall myocardial oxygen consumption and in clinical practice the situation is further complicated by interaction between the major determinants of MVO_2:

1. *MVO_2 of the non-beating heart*
   Basal myocardial metabolism accounts for 25% of the myocardial oxygen demand.

2. *Wall tension*
   At a fixed heart rate myocardial wall tension is the major determinant of MVO_2. Stress develops when tension is applied to a cross sectional area (Laplace):

$$\text{Wall stress} = \frac{\text{pressure} \times \text{radius}}{2 \times \text{wall thickness}}$$

Table 7.1

Determinants of myocardial oxygen demand
1. MVO_2 of the non-beating heart
2. Wall tension (diastolic volume, ventricular pressure)
3. Heart rate
4. Contractility

Determinants of myocardial oxygen supply
1. Myocardial blood flow
2. Arterial oxygen content (CaO_2)
3. Diffusion distances (capillary arrangement and reserve)
4. Oxygen dissociation curve (HbP_{50})

In a clinical setting the calculation of wall stress is impracticable as a routine procedure; however, two major determinants of wall stress can be measured, namely the left ventricular filling pressure ('preload') and the systemic vascular resistance ('afterload') using a thermodilution (Swan-Ganz) balloon flotation catheter (see Ch. 20).

3. *Heart rate*

An increase in heart rate increases MVO_2 due to an inherent associated increase in the force of contraction (the staircase phenomenon or treppe), in addition coronary perfusion is reduced due to the shortened diastole.

4. *Contractility*

Alterations in contractility (or the force-velocity relationship) alter MVO_2 independent of the effects of wall tension or heart rate.

PRINCIPLES OF VASODILATOR THERAPY

The cardiovascular system responds to myocardial failure in a number of ways. Firstly the ventricle dilates which initially facilitates an increase in stroke volume by the Starling mechanism. However, in patients with heart failure the Starling curve is rather flat such that changes in 'preload' are less important than in the normal subject (Fig. 7.1); thus a further increase in 'preload' merely increases wall stress (hence MVO_2) without

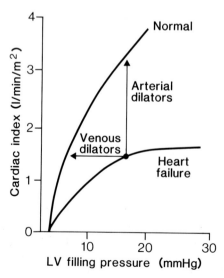

Fig. 7.1 Principles of vasodilator therapy

any appreciable increase in stroke volume. Vasodilator therapy aims to reduce 'preload' to such a level that wall stress is reduced without adversely affecting stroke volume.

In response to a low cardiac output a reflex rise in arterial pressure occurs in an attempt to maintain tissue perfusion. Systemic vascular resistance increases as a result of an increase in circulating angiotensin II and catecholamines. The failing heart is particularly sensitive to alterations in systemic vascular resistance; a reduction in systemic vascular resistance ('afterload') will reduce arterial blood pressure (hence wall stress) as well as lead to an increase in cardiac output.

Classification of the vasodilators

Vasodilators can act at three sites:
1. *Venous dilators*
   Pure venous dilators (e.g. nitrates) reduce an elevated ventricular filling pressure without changing cardiac output. Consequently, the reduction in pulmonary venous pressure relieves pulmonary oedema; left ventricular volume and wall stress are reduced and the reduction in left ventricular end diastolic pressure increases coronary perfusion pressure.
2. *Arterial dilators*
   Arteriolar dilators (e.g. hydrallazine) lower systemic vascular resistance and increase cardiac output for any given filling pressure. In addition, a fall in left ventricular systolic pressure reduces MVO$_2$. Arterial vasodilators may also be used with benefit in systemic hypertension (see Ch. 4), mitral and aortic regurgitation (see Chs. 8 and 9 respectively).
3. *Combination vasodilators*
   Using a combination of arterial and venous dilators or an agent which acts at both sites (e.g. nitroprusside) load reduction can be optimised for an individual patient.

Specific agents

Doses are listed in Table 7.2.

Venous dilators
Nitrates
Predominately venous dilators with little arterial action. An increase in venous capacitance causes a reduction in 'preload' and hence ventricular volume and MVO$_2$. A reduction in LVEDP facilitates subendocardial blood flow. Nitrates may be administered by the sublingual, oral, intravenous and transcutaneous routes (see p. 15, Table 1.7). Sublingual nitrates are usually reserved for the patient with angina pectoris where the rapid absorption and short duration of action (peak blood level 2 minutes, half-life 7 minutes) are ideal. Long-acting oral nitrates or transcutaneous nitrates are used for chronic vasodilator therapy, usually

Table 7.2 Vasodilator drugs and doses

	Route	Daily Dose	Dose frequency
Venous dilators			
Nitrates	IV, PO	see page 15	
Frusemide	IV, PO	20–250 mg	12–24 hourly
Arterial dilators			
Hydrallazine	PO	75–200 mg	6–8 hourly
Diazeoxide	PO	400–1000 mg	8–12 hourly
Minoxidil	PO	5–50 mg	12–24 hourly
Phentolamine	IV	0.1–2 mg/min	infusion
Indoramin	PO	50–200 mg	12–24 hourly
Isoprenaline	IV	0.5–10 μg/min	infusion
Salbutamol	PO	see page 134	infusion
Calcium antagonists	PO	see page 19	
Trimetaphan	IV	from 3–4 mg/min	infusion
Combined vasodilators			
Nitroprusside	IV	10–200 μg/min	infusion
Prazosin	PO	2–20 mg	8–12 hourly
Captopril	PO	18.75–150 mg	8–12 hourly
Enalapril	PO	5–20 mg	12–24 hourly

in combination with an arterial dilator. Nitrates used alone may cause a tachycardia and reflex vasoconstriction. After a run in period other side-effects (e.g. headache) are uncommon and tachyphylaxis and cross-tolerance is rare. In some patients with mitral regurgitation nitrates may adversely affect forward output. Nitrates are discussed in more detail in Chapter 1.

Frusemide
Intravenous frusemide is a weak venodilator. This secondary effect of the drug accounts for the subjective improvement in patients with pulmonary oedema prior to the onset of a diuresis.

Arterial dilators
1. Direct vasodilators (smooth muscle relaxants)

   Hydrallazine
   Arteriolar dilator with probable direct inotropic action. Rapidly absorbed from the gut (peak blood levels 1–2 h, half-life 2–8 h), but the therapeutic action is prolonged due to binding in the arterial wall. Acetylated in the liver and excreted in the urine. Improved renal blood flow may augment response to diuretics. Absence of reflex tachycardia in patients with heart failure may be due to down-regulation of adrenergic receptors in this group. Specific tachyphylaxis develops after 6 months treatment in most patients and is the major problem in treating the patient with cardiac failure. 5–10% of patients develop a reversible lupus-like syndrome which is particularly common in patients treated with 200 mg or more of the drug per day. Drug induced lupus is more common in white patients, females, slow acetylators and

carriers of the HLA type DR4. Although positive antinuclear antibodies develop in 30–60% all patients after three years treatment, the incidence of the syndrome is only 1–3% overall. Other side effects include nausea, headache and gastrointestinal disturbance.

Diazoxide

Protein bound arterial vasodilator with an ill-sustained vasodilator action. Side effects include tachycardia, diabetes mellitus, fluid retention (renin release). Used for accelerated hypertension (see Ch. 4).

Minoxidil

Arterial vasodilator with a prolonged half-life of 1–4 days. Poorly tolerated due to hirsutism, tachycardia and fluid retention. Pericardial effusion has also been reported. Occasionally used for resistant systemic hypertension (see Ch. 4) but unsuitable as a vasodilator.

2. Alpha antagonists

Phentolamine

Blocks both pre-synaptic (alpha$_1$) and post-synaptic (alpha$_2$) receptors to cause arterial vasodilatation. Phentolamine is also a weak peripheral beta agonist, and the mild inotropic action may be due to noradrenaline release. Due to a short half-life phentolamine is used almost exclusively as an intravenous infusion when it results in a reduction in systemic vascular resistance and an increase in cardiac output. Phentolamine is a weak venodilator with little effect on ventricular filling pressure. Side effects include diarrhoea, tachycardia and exacerbation of angina.

Indoramin

Selective alpha$_1$ antagonist with membrane stabilising activity; also antagonises the actions of histamine and serotonin. Little data on the use of indoramin as a vasodilator. Extensive protein binding and first-pass hepatic metabolism. Side effects include sedation, failure to ejaculate, dry mouth, depression and fluid retention.

3. Beta agonists

Isoprenaline

Pure beta (beta$_1$ and beta$_2$) agonist. Causes an increase in heart rate and contractility (beta$_1$) and hence MVO_2. Arterial vasodilatation causes a reduction in 'afterload' due to the beta$_2$ effect. Reduction in pulmonary vascular resistance is particularly useful in pulmonary hypertension (e.g. immediately following mitral valve replacement). Side effects include ventricular and atrial arrhythmias and systemic hypotension.

Salbutamol

Selective beta$_2$ agonist causing arterial vasodilatation, a reduction in systemic vascular resistance and an increase in cardiac output. Little or no increase in contractility (or MVO$_2$). Possible direct vasodilator action on the coronary circulation. Side effects including tachycardia similar to isoprenaline.

4. Calcium antagonists

Verapamil

Reduces systemic vascular resistance and mean arterial blood pressure with little or no change in cardiac output. Negative inotropic action may be troublesome in patients with impaired ventricular function. Used for the treatment of angina pectoris (see Ch. 1) and as an antiarrhythmic agent (see Ch. 16)

Nifedipine

Arterial vasodilator with a mild venodilator action. No significant increase in heart rate but fluid retention may have an adverse effect in patients with heart failure. Acute pulmonary oedema has been precipitated by nifedipine in occasional patients with coronary artery disease. Other side effects include nausea, dizziness, headache and facial flushing. Mainly used for the treatment of angina pectoris (see Ch. 1) and in systemic hypertension (see Ch. 4).

Diltiazem

Little data available in patients with heart failure. Appears to be a weaker vasodilator than nifedipine and less depressant than verapamil.

5. Ganglion blocking drugs

Trimetaphan

Administered as an intravenous infusion. Blocks neural transmission at autonomic ganglia; predominantly an arteriolar dilator with secondary action on venous capacitance vessels. Degree of pre-existing sympathetic tone determines the degree of systemic hypotension. Tachyphylaxis may occur. Side effects include tachycardia, postural hypotension, mydriasis, cycloplegia, anhidrosis, urinary retention and constipation. Glomerular filtration rate may be reduce in normotensive subjects. Use with care in patients with a history of allergy as trimetaphan stimulates histamine release.

Combined vasodilators

Nitroprusside

Balanced arterial and venodilator. Used as an intravenous infusion and titrated against the systemic blood pressure. Haemodynamic response starts within minutes and stops almost immediately the infusion is discontinued. Free cyanide is liberated in tissues and red cells and converted into thiocyanate by the enzyme rhodanase in the liver. Excretion is renal with a half-life of one week. Toxicity may develop after 48 hours treatment if thiocyanate levels exceed 100 μg/ml and may be prevented by administration of hydroxycobalamin. Side effects include fatigue, nausea, anorexia, disorientation, muscle spasms and rarely hypothyroidism. In clinical practice dosage is limited by systemic hypotension.

Prazosin

Haemodynamic equivalent to 'oral nitroprusside'. A quinazoline derivative that selectively blocks alpha$_1$ sites in both arteries and veins producing balanced vasodilatation. Preservation of the alpha$_2$ activity reduces reflex tachycardia. Prazosin undergoes first pass liver metabolism with 50–70% reaching the systemic circulation unchanged. High (95%) protein binding causes a three to four fold increase in the concentration of active drug in hypoalbuminaemia. Plasma half-life 3–4 hours, but prolonged clinical effect means that twice daily oral dosing is appropriate for most patients. Hepatic metabolism and elimination in the faeces. Specific tachyphylaxis to prazosin may develop over 2–6 months therapy, but there is some evidence to indicate that the attenuation of the long-term response may be related to an excessive reduction in 'preload' by additional diuretic therapy, or alternatively a true blunting of the dose-response curve. The drug is generally well tolerated; side effects include the first-dose phenomenon (see p. 85), headache, drowsiness, depression, nasal congestion, impotence and incontinence.

Converting enzyme inhibitors (Captopril, Enalapril)

Captopril was the first available orally active inhibitor of angiotensin converting enzyme (ACE). ACE is responsible for converting angiotensin I to the potent vasoconstrictor angiotensin II (or kininase II) which also stimulates aldosterone secretion (and hence sodium retention) by the distal tubule via the adrenal cortex. Acute studies indicate that Captopril reduces systemic vascular resistance with little change in heart rate, cardiac output or pulmonary capillary wedge pressure. During long-term treatment variable changes in cardiac output may occur suggesting an additional action on venous capacitance vessels, although captopril appears not to interfere with normal baroreceptor reflexes. Captopril is rapidly absorbed by mouth with an effect occurring as soon as 10 minutes after ingestion and peak levels within one hour. Approximately 75% of the administered dose is absorbed during fasting and this may be reduced by 30–40% when the drug is taken with food. Although the half-life appears to be less than two hours, clinical effects do not correlate with plasma levels, and three times daily dosing is recommended unless the creatinine clearance is less than 75 ml/min in which case the drug should be given less frequently.

Low initial doses (e.g. 6.25 mg three times daily) are appropriate when Captopril is used as a vasodilator, and the dose of concomitant diuretic therapy may need to be reduced in order to avoid severe systemic hypotension. If the initial dose is tolerated then the dose can be doubled every few days up to approximately 50 mg three times daily.

PRACTICAL APPROACH TO VASODILATOR THERAPY

The practical approach to the use of vasodilators is similar whether myocardial impairment is due to acute myocardial infarction, dilated cardiomyopathy or chronic aortic regurgitation. The patient is carefully assessed to determine whether the major problem is an elevation in pulmonary venous pressure resulting in breathlessness, or a reduction in cardiac output, reduced tissue perfusion and an elevation in systemic vascular resistance causing fatigue and general malaise.

In an acute situation accurate monitoring of 'preload', 'afterload' and cardiac output by a flow-directed (Swan-Ganz) thermodilution catheter inserted at the bedside (see Ch. 20) is a prerequisite to the appropriate management of intravenous fluids and vasodilator therapy. Furthermore, the finding of a low PACWP indicates that the patient is suffering from intravascular depletion, hence requiring fluid replenishment rather than vasodilators. An outline of the appropriate management of vasodilator therapy depending on the haemodynamics is shown in Table 7.3

In patients with chronic left ventricular dysfunction symptoms are due to a combination of an elevated pulmonary vascular resistance, a low

Table 7.3 Haemodynamics and management of patients with impaired myocardial function

PACW pressure	Systemic BP	Cardiac index	Management
Low	Low	Normal	Volume
Low	Low	Low	Volume
Normal	Normal	Low	Arterial dilators
Normal	Low	Low	Inotropes ± arterial dilators
High	Normal	Low	Venous dilators
High	Low	Low	Inotropes ± venous dilators

Normal PACW pressure (mean) = 8–12 mm Hg
Normal cardiac index = 3.0 + 0.5 litres/min/m^2

cardiac output and an elevated systemic vascular resistance. In the majority of cases a predominantly arterial dilator with a secondary venodilator action (e.g. Captopril, Enalapril) is appropriate. Oral nitrates (e.g. Isosorbide mononitrate) can be added if an additional reduction in pulmonary venous pressure is required.

Despite advances in the understanding and development of vasodilator therapy there is as yet little data to indicate that long-term prognosis is improved in patients with impaired myocardial function. The one year mortality in patients with symptoms at rest or on mild exertion is 40–50%.

8. MITRAL VALVE DISEASE

MITRAL STENOSIS

Stenosis of the mitral valve is a late consequence of rheumatic carditis. Isolated mitral stenosis accounts for 40% of cases of rheumatic valve disease and involvement of the aortic valve without concomitant mitral disease is rare. A previous history of acute rheumatic fever can be obtained in only 50% of patients. Females are affected more frequently than males (2–3:1). A latency period of 20 years between the acute infection and symptomatic valvular dysfunction is not uncommon with the typical patient presenting in the fourth or fifth decade. In immigrants (e.g. from the Middle East, Asia and South America) severe valvular disease may be present by the early twenties. Mitral stenosis may rarely occur as a congenital anomaly, usually in association with other congenital heart defects.

Pathophysiology

The mitral valve is a bicuspid valve consisting of a larger anterior cusp and a smaller posterior cusp supported by approximately 120 fibrous chordae tendineae which are attached to two papillary muscles. The normal mitral valve has a cross-sectional area of 4–5 cm² which is reduced to 1 cm² or less when stenosis is critical. At rest, blood flows through the normal mitral valve at approximately 150 ml/s during diastole, and even when flow increases at times of increased cardiac output (e.g. on exercise) no significant gradient is generated between the left atrium and left ventricle.

Mitral stenosis cannot be regarded as a discrete obstruction to left ventricular inflow because the rheumatic process affects the mitral sub-valve apparatus resulting in chordal fusion, shortening and tethering. Thus, calculations of mitral valve area either using haemodynamic parameters or directly by cross-sectional echocardiography have limited application.

The majority of ventricular filling occurs in the first third of diastole (rapid filling phase) and during the last third of diastole (atrial systole). During the period of diastasis in mid-diastole there is little or no forward

138

flow and the mitral valve may actually close. In sinus rhythm, atrial systole contributes approximately 20% of the cardiac output. The importance of ventricular rate, hence the duration of diastole, as a determinant of the transmitral gradient cannot be overstated; this, together with the loss of atrial transport accounts for the dramatic symptomatic deterioration that accompanies the onset of atrial fibrillation in these patients.

Mitral stenosis is frequently associated with a degree of regurgitation; mitral regurgitation predominates in only 35% of cases.

Symptoms

Clinical features of mitral stenosis are determined by the left atrial pressure, the cardiac output and the pulmonary vascular resistance.

Increased left atrial pressure

1. *Breathlessness*

   With the increase in left atrial and pulmonary venous pressure, fluid increases in the interstitium of the lung which reduces pulmonary compliance and increases the work of breathing. Changes in interstitial pressure also alter the closing volume of small airways which is detrimental to efficient pulmonary function.

   When mitral stenosis is mild (mitral valve area 2.5 cm^2) breathlessness only occurs at times of increased cardiac output (e.g. stress, fever, exercise, pregnancy, surgery) and is usually insidious. An abrupt reduction in exercise tolerance may complicate the onset of atrial fibrillation with a rapid ventricular rate.

   As the severity of the mitral lesion increases the patient experiences breathlessness on lying flat (orthopnoea). Orthopnoea is due to the increase in venous return, an increase in hydrostatic pressure in the upper zones of the lungs and a reduction in vital capacity that accompanies the change in posture. Chronic pulmnoary disease may also cause orthopnoea, as may any other cause of increased left atrial pressure (e.g. dilated cardiomyopathy). Later still the patient may experience nocturnal coughing or nocturnal dyspnoea as the pulmonary venous pressure increases still further (see Ch. 5).

2. *Haemoptysis*

   A number of types of haemoptysis are recognised in mitral stenosis including blood streaked sputum, frothy pink sputum, haemoptysis complicating pulmonary embolism and rarely a brisk haemoptysis caused by rupture of a dilated pulmonary vein (pulmonary apoplexy).

3. *Bronchitis*
Up to 30% of patients with moderate to severe mitral stenosis experience recurrent bronchitis. It has been suggested that respiratory infection results from excessive mucus production complicating bronchial hyperaemia.

Pulmonary hypertension

With increasing degrees of mitral stenosis, pulmonary arterial pressure rises in parallel with left atrial pressure (passive pulmonary hypertension). In most patients mean PA pressure is 10–12 mmHg greater than mean LA pressure. In some patients, particularly those with severe mitral stenosis, pulmonary arterial pressure rises disproportionately (reactive pulmonary hypertension). The development of severe PHT is unpredictable in an individual patient but may be due to reflex pulmonary arteriolar vasoconstriction, an increase in pulmonary arteriolar tone secondary to hypoxia, or a reduction in the effective pulmonary vascular bed by fibrosis, embolism or infarction.

1. *Fatigue*
Low cardiac output complicating pulmonary hypertension causes fatigue and lethargy due to the reduction in cerebral and musculoskeletal perfusion.

2. *Anorexia*
An increase in central venous pressure causes hepatic and gut congestion resulting in loss of appetite, abdominal pain, malabsorption and weight loss. In extreme cases breathlessness itself may make eating difficult.

3. *Fluid retention*
Peripheral oedema and abdominal distension complicate right heart failure.

Complications of mitral stenosis

1. *Palpitations*
Atrial fibrillation occurs in 40% of patients with mitral stenosis, and the incidence increases with advancing age and an increase in left atrial dimension. By the age of 50 years, 80% of patients are in atrial fibrillation. Ventricular arrhythmias are uncommon.

2. *Systemic embolism*
Symptoms related to systemic embolism occur in 15–20% of patients with significant mitral stenosis. Any major artery may be involved, but cerebral emboli are particularly common accounting for 60–70% of the total. Atrial fibrillation, increasing age and the size of the LA appendage are all related to the incidence of systemic embolism. Right atrial thrombus may lead to pulmonary embolism. Prior to the advent of valve surgery, 20% of deaths were attributable to thromboembolism.

3. *Infective endocarditis*
In uncomplicated mitral stenosis, infective endocarditis is rare and accounts for only 5–10% of deaths in medically treated series. Infection is more common in mixed mitral valve disease or when there is additional aortic involvement.

4. *Chest pain*
5–10% of patients experience chest pain typical of myocardial ischaemia. Although a coronary embolism may be responsible in some patients, the aetiology remains obscure in the majority.

Physical signs

1. *Facies*
So-called mitral facies (malar flush) is due to a low cardiac output causing peripheral cyanosis and usually indicates severe disease associated with pulmonary hypertension. The finding is non-specific.

2. *Pulse*
Normal unless severe pulmonary hypertension has caused a fall in cardiac output. Atrial fibrillation is common.

3. *Venous pressure*
Pulmonary hypertension is accompanied by a prominent 'a' wave. In atrial fibrillation the 'a' wave is absent, and a systolic ('cv') wave accompanies secondary tricuspid regurgitation.

4. *Precordial impulse*
Typically the heart is not enlarged. S1 may be palpable to the left of the sternum ('tapping apex'); pulmonary hypertension causes a left parasternal heave (from the RV) and P2 may be palpated in the second left intercostal space. On turning the patient onto the left side a diastolic thrill may be palpable over the apex if the murmur is loud.

5. *Heart sounds and murmurs*
A loud S1 due to closure of the rheumatic mitral valve is the most important sign in mitral stenosis and should alert the clinician to a careful search for a diastolic murmur — particularly if the patient is in atrial fibrillation. Rarely, in severe calcific mitral stenosis S1 can be normal and if the cardiac output is low the diastolic murmur is inaudible because of low forward flow. P2 is loud in pulmonary hypertension, and in severe PHT S2 may become single. Sudden tensing of the mitral leaflets by the subvalve apparatus and the halting of the downward movement of the mitral valve causes a high pitched opening snap (OS) best heard between the left sternal border and the cardiac apex 40–120 ms after S2. It occurs later than P2 and earlier than

an S3 (which is never present in isolated mitral stenosis). The S2-OS interval varies inversely with mean LA pressure as long as the valve has some mobility. An opening snap can be heard in 90% of patients with mitral stenosis.

In mild stenosis the low pitched rumbling diastolic murmur is short and mid-diastolic in timing and well localised to the apex radiating to the axilla. The length not the loudness of the murmur relates to the severity of the lesion. Presystolic accentuation is classically described in sinus rhythm, but if the valve is mobile it may occasionally be present in atrial fibrillation. Turning the patient onto the left side, expiration or mild exercise will all accentuate the murmur. Other murmurs that may be present include a pansystolic murmur in tricuspid regurgitation and the Graham Steell murmur of pulmonary regurgitation.

6. *Lungs*

In moderate or severe disease the signs of pulmonary oedema may be obvious (see Ch. 5).

7. *Abdominal examination*

Hepatic enlargement (which may be pulsatile), ascites and peripheral oedema accompany pulmonary hypertension, tricuspid regurgitation and an elevated venous pressure.

Investigations

1. *Electrocardiography*

In patients in sinus rhythm left atrial enlargement is detected by a wide P wave (>120 ms in lead II), which is biphasic in V_1 (P mitrale) — both these features are non-specific (e.g. also occur in LV disease) but are present in 90% of patients with significant mitral stenosis. P wave morphology is related to LA volume rather than LA pressure. 40% of patients are in atrial fibrillation; the size of the fibrillation waves relate neither to left atrial volume or pressure. With the development of pulmonary hypertension there are features of right ventricular hypertrophy (right axis deviation, right bundle branch block, R:S>1 in V_1), followed by right atrial enlargement (P pulmonale).

2. *Chest radiograph*

In pure mitral stenosis the cardiothoracic ratio is normal unless pulmonary hypertension has caused right ventricular dilatation. The left atrium is selectively enlarged causing elevation of the left main bronchus (more easily seen on a penetrated film). Mitral valve calcification may be seen on the lateral projection and confirmed by fluoroscopy. In the elderly this must be differentiated from mitral annulus calcification (see p. 150). With elevation in left atrial pressure, pulmonary venous distension occurs followed by upper lobe blood diversion and the radiographic signs of acute pulmonary oedema (see Ch. 5). In pulmonary hypertension the proximal pulmonary arteries are dilated and there may be peripheral pruning. Pulmonary haemosiderosis and ossification rarely occur in association with long-standing disease.

3. *M-mode and cross-sectional echocardiography*
   Echocardiography is the single most useful investigation in mitral stenosis, and in some centres mitral valve surgery is undertaken on the basis of the physical examination together with a detailed echocardiographic assessment without cardiac catheterisation. Furthermore, suitability for a conservative procedure (e.g. valvotomy) is best determined by echocardiography. The features of mitral stenosis seen on the M-mode are listed in Table 8.1. Typical cases show a thickened mitral valve with a reduction in the mid-diastolic closure rate of the anterior leaflet. The posterior cusp is also reduced in mobility and moves anteriorly (instead of posteriorly) during diastole. The left atrial dimension is increased and thrombus may be visible in the left atrial appendage on the cross-sectional image. Analysis of the left ventricular filling pattern is the most sensitive means of assessing the severity of the valve lesion; in significant mitral stenosis the normal rapid filling phase followed by diastasis is lost — filling is reduced in rate and prolonged in time.

4. *Doppler*
   Pressure drop detected across the mitral valve using continuous wave Doppler correlates well with the gradient measured at catheterisation. As with haemodynamic assessment of the mitral gradient, changes in heart rate may alter the gradient detected by Doppler. If the cardiac output is low the Doppler gradient may be inaccurate; in this case the pressure half-time may be more reliable and is related to the mitral valve area.

5. *Haemodynamics*
   Invasive assessment of the patient with mitral valve disease is only required in certain circumstances (table 8.2).

Table 8.1 M-mode echocardiographic features of mitral stenosis

1. Reduced mitral closing velocity (EF slope)
2. Anterior movement of the posterior mitral leaflet during diastole
3. Diminished separation of the anterior and posterior mitral leaflets
4. Thickening of the mitral leaflets
5. Reduced left ventricular filling rate
6. Loss of rapid filling and diastasis during ventricular diastole

Table 8.2 Indications for cardiac catheterisation in patients with mitral stenosis

1. Confirmation of the severity of the mitral valve lesion or assessment of left ventricular function in a patient who is not echogenic
2. Calculation of the pulmonary vascular resistance
3. Assessment of concomitant aortic valve disease
4. Exclusion of additional coronary artery disease

The mitral valve gradient, mitral valve area and pulmonary vascular resistance can be calculated using standard formulae (Ch. 21). Formerly, patients with a very high pulmonary vascular resistance (>10 Wood units) were not accepted for operation. With modern surgical and anaesthetic techniques this is now not the case although the preoperative PVR is a major determinant of the symptomatic benefit following mitral valve surgery. Changes in haemodynamics occurring during exercise give additional information as to the severity of the mitral lesion.

6. *Cineangiography*
   Left ventricular function is evaluated by recording cineangiograms in the standard projections, and a semiquantitative assessment of the severity of additional mitral regurgitation can also be made. Left atrial size is best determined by echocardiography. In selected patients (e.g. males over 40 years, patients with a history of chest pain) coronary arteriography is carried out using conventional techniques (Ch. 20).

7. *Other tests*
   Respiratory function testing should be undertaken prior to considering mitral valve surgery as concomitant airflow obstruction may be a significant factor in reducing exercise tolerance.

   Hyperthyroidism should always be considered in the symptomatic patient with apparently mild stenosis because the associated tachycardia is poorly tolerated.

Differential diagnosis

1. *Atrial myxoma*
   Rare. May mimic mitral stenosis in all respects. Patients present with constitutional disturbance, loss of consciousness, systemic emboli and changing murmurs. Atrial myxoma can be excluded with certainty by echocardiography which reveals the characteristic mass of echoes behind the posterior mitral leaflet in diastole.

2. *Cor triatriatum*
   Very rare. A third atrium that receives the pulmonary veins and is separated from the true left atrium by a membrane. Easily recognised by echocardiography.

3. *Atrial septal defect*

The wrong interpretation of physical signs may occasionally lead to diagnostic confusion between a secundum ASD and mitral stenosis. In an ASD, S2 is widely split with a delay in the pulmonary component, but a mid-diastolic tricuspid flow murmur preceded by a tricuspid opening snap may mimic mitral stenosis. The two lesions may rarely coexist (Lutembacher's syndrome).

4. *Austin Flint murmur*

The regurgitant jet in aortic regurgitation causes vibration of the anterior leaflet of the mitral valve resulting in a mid-diastolic murmur (Austin Flint murmur) indistinguishable from mitral stenosis. Other features of aortic regurgitation are listed in Chapter 9; the normal S1 and absent mitral opening snap assist in the correct interpretation of the physical signs, which can be confirmed by echocardiography.

Natural history of mitral stenosis

Patients with mitral stenosis usually become symptomatic 10–20 years after acute rheumatic fever. A progressive deterioration from mild to severe disability occurs over a 5–10 year period. Prior to the advent of cardiac surgery 20% of patients were dead 5 years after starting medical treatment and 40% had died after 10 years. Congestive cardiac failure accounted for 60% of deaths and thromboembolism 20%.

Medical management

1. *Digoxin*

In patients in atrial fibrillation the ventricular rate is controlled with oral digoxin at a dose sufficient to maintain the resting rate at 60–80/min (0.0625–0.25 mg once daily depending on age, weight and renal function). There is no place for 'prophylactic' digoxin for the patient in sinus rhythm because this course of action does not control the ventricular rate at the onset of atrial fibrillation. Occasional patients require additional beta blocking drugs (e.g. Propranolol 10–20 mg twice daily) or calcium antagonists (e.g. Verapamil 40 mg three times daily) to control rate, but difficulty in controlling the ventricular rate may indicate that the severity of the mitral valve lesion has been underestimated. Frequently, digoxin does not control exercise induced tachycardia.

Cardioversion is rarely successful in restoring sinus rhythm in the patient with mitral stenosis except perhaps the young patient in atrial fibrillation who has undergone mitral valvotomy and was in sinus rhythm preoperatively. Any patient with mitral stenosis who is cardioverted should be previously anticoagulated with warfarin as the risk of thromboembolism without anticoagulants is 1–2%.

2. *Diuretics*
Fluid retention responds to diuretics but they are of limited efficacy in pulmonary oedema as this will have resulted from a fixed anatomical obstruction. Over vigorous diuretic therapy results in hypovolaemia and pre-renal azotaemia. Thiazide and combination diuretics are more appropriate than large doses of loop diuretics.

3. *Anticoagulation*
In view of the risks of thromboembolism, all patients with mitral stenosis who are in atrial fibrillation should be anticoagulated with warfarin to maintain the British corrected prothrombin ratio between 2.5 and 3.3 times the control value. Patients over the age of 35 years are prone to develop systemic emboli and should be anticoagulated even if they are in sinus rhythm. Up to 30% of emboli in mitral stenosis occur in patients in sinus rhythm. In elderly patients (>70 years) without a previous history of thromboembolism the risk of anticoagulation probably exceeds the potential benefit.

4. *Antibiotics*
Despite the low incidence of infective endocarditis in mitral stenosis, all patients should receive antibiotic prophylaxis for dental and operative procedures and other potentially septic hazards (see Ch. 11).

Surgery in mitral stenosis

The decision to perform surgery in patients with mitral stenosis is not determined by the mitral gradient or a particular mitral valve area but by symptoms and exercise tolerance. Other indications for surgery are listed in Table 8.3.

The long-term results of mitral valve surgery are less favourable than those of aortic valve replacement and this should always be considered especially as symptomatic deterioration may be very slow in mitral valve disease. Furthermore, a conservative mitral procedure can never be guaranteed and for this reason the results of valve replacement are relevant to all patients undergoing mitral valve surgery, even if the intention is to perform mitral valvotomy or repair.

Table 8.3 Indications for surgery in mitral stenosis

1. Limiting symptoms and a reduced exercise tolerance
2. Severe pulmonary hypertension
3. Recurrent emboli despite adequate anticoagulation
4. Intended pregnancy

Mitral valvotomy

1. Closed valvotomy

Mitral valvotomy remains an excellent operation in selected cases and is feasible in approximately 70% of patients with pure mitral stenosis. It is not appropriate if there is severe valve calcification or when the rheumatic process has destroyed much of the sub-valve apparatus leading to mitral regurgitation. Closed valvotomy using a dilator introduced through the left atrial appendage has been successfully used for many years, but the number of surgeons experienced in the procedure is decreasing. The early mortality of closed mitral valvotomy is 1–2%, the early embolic rate 6%. Late systemic embolism even without anticoagulation is uncommon (approximately 1% per patient-year follow-up) — presumably due to removal of the left atrial appendage at the time of operation. Symptomatic improvement is excellent in most patients. Within 15 years of mitral valvotomy, symptomatic restenosis occurs in approximately 30% of patients; this subgroup will require reoperation, usually mitral valve replacement.

2. Open valvotomy

Despite having to be undertaken on cardiopulmonary bypass, open valvotomy allows the mitral valve to be split under direct vision and additional procedures can be carried out on the sub-valve apparatus if necessary. Furthermore, if the valvotomy is technically unsatisfactory the patient can proceed to mitral valve replacement at the same operation. The early mortality from open mitral valvotomy is 1–2%.

Mitral valve replacement

Mitral valve replacement is appropriate for patients with symptomatic mitral stenosis who are not suitable for mitral valvotomy. Valve replacement may be undertaken using a mechanical valve of the tilting-disc type (e.g. Bjork-Shiley) or ball type (e.g. Starr-Edwards), or alternatively a tissue valve (e.g. Carpentier-Edwards porcine xenograft). All prosthetic valves have a measurable diastolic gradient of 2–5 mmHg which may rise to 5–15 mmHg on exercise; thus, a mitral prosthesis is itself mildly stenotic.

Early mortality for mitral valve replacement is 6–8% and is not related to the type of valve used. Elderly patients and those with a very large left atrium, severe pulmonary hypertension or additional coronary artery disease fare less well.

The choice of prosthesis is determined by the surgeon and the particular patient. For example, a low profile valve (e.g. Bjork-Shiley) may be appropriate for the patient with a small left ventricle. All mechanical valves require anticoagulation with warfarin which may be difficult to manage in the elderly and pregnant patients. The incidence of thromboembolic complications is similar in the two types of mechanical valves (3–5% per patient-year), although disc valves tend to thrombose in situ and ball valves result in systemic emboli. Complications of anticoagulation account for a further 2–4% per patient-year. However the incidence of valve failure with mechanical valves is very low (2% per patient-year).

Long-term durability of tissue valves is less certain although they have the advantage that anticoagulants are only continued for 2–3 months after operation in most series. The effects of chronic atrial fibrillation on the incidence of late thromboembolism following mitral valve replacement with tissue valves has not been fully resolved. Thromboembolic complications occur at a rate of 1–2% per patient-year. Tissue degeneration leading to valve failure has an acceptably low incidence of approximately 2% per patient-year for the first 5–6 years, but this gradually increases such that the probability of operation or death from this complication reaches 20% by 9 years. Tissue valves are unsuitable for children or young adults (<20 years) as the incidence of premature calcification is unacceptable (30–50% at five years).

The overall late mortality for all patients undergoing mitral valve replacement of 3–5% per annum and is similar for all currently available valves.

ACUTE MITRAL REGURGITATION

Acute mitral regurgitation should be regarded as functionally distinct from chronic mitral regurgitation. Sudden mitral regurgitation may be caused by destruction of the valve by endocarditis (cusp perforation or chordal rupture), papillary muscle rupture (partial or total) complicating acute myocardial infarction (see Ch. 2), or spontaneous chordal rupture.

Unlike the situation in chronic mitral regurgitation there is insufficient time for compensatory mechanisms to adapt to the volume load. Both the left ventricle and left atrium are normal in size. Acute pulmonary oedema occurs early and without surgical intervention death occurs in 75% of patients within 48 hours.

Appropriate management consists of correction of arterial hypoxaemia with ventilation and positive end expiratory pressure if necessary, exclusion of active infection (see Ch. 11), and early valve replacement or repair. Arterial vasodilators (e.g. Nitroprusside) have a limited role in the preoperative period (see Ch. 7).

CHRONIC NON-RHEUMATIC MITRAL REGURGITATION

Chronic mitral regurgitation is one of the most difficult types of valvular heart disease to manage appropriately. The natural history of the condition is prolonged and the haemodynamic consequences are well tolerated. Many patients require no specific treatment. In others, if operative intervention is unduly delayed irreversible myocardial damage results in a poor symptomatic result.

Aetiology

There are numerous causes of chronic mitral regurgitation. Pure mitral regurgitation as a consequence of chronic rheumatic disease is rare; most often there is mixed mitral valve disease. Causes of chronic non-rheumatic mitral regurgitation are listed in Table 8.4.

1. *'Floppy' mitral valve*

   May occur in isolation or as part of the mitral valve prolapse syndrome (see p. 155). A spectrum of valve abnormality ranging from minor degrees of cusp overlap (present in 5–15% of the population), to a 'floppy' valve causing significant mitral regurgitation. In the more severe forms a hereditary disorder of collagen synthesis leads to redundant cusp tissue, chordal attenuation and rupture.

2. *Dilated mitral annulus*

   A dilated annulus in isolation as a cause of mitral regurgitation is rare. Left ventricular end-diastolic volume has to become very large to cause passive dilatation of the annulus. Most cases of mitral regurgitation attributed to annular dilatation are caused by abnormal papillary muscle geometry.

3. *(Partial) chordal rupture*

   Rupture of a few chordae result in chronic mitral regurgitation which may progress as a result of further chordal rupture. Chordae are avascular and it is likely that chordal rupture is due to myxomatous degeneration rather than ischaemia. Posterior chordal rupture is more frequent than anterior rupture. Spontaneous rupture may occur in a 'floppy' mitral valve and the two conditions frequently coexist.

4. *Papillary muscle dysfunction*

   Caused by ischaemia of one or both papillary muscles, or by dilatation of the left ventricular cavity. Integrity of the mitral valve is dependent on contraction of the papillary muscles. Each papillary muscle is supplied by an end-artery, and the posterior papillary muscle (supplied by the right coronary artery) is particularly susceptible to ischaemia. Dilatation of

Table 8.4 Causes of non-rheumatic mitral regurgitation

1. 'Floppy' mitral valve
2. Dilated mitral annulus
3. (Partial) chordal rupture
4. Papillary muscle dysfunction
5. Mitral annulus calcification
6. Infective endocarditis
7. Hypertrophic cardiomyopathy
8. Connective tissue disease (e.g. Marfan's syndrome, pseudoxanthoma elasticum, osteogenesis imperfecta)
9. Congenital defects (mitral cleft, parachute valve)

the left ventricle alters the spatial relationship of the papillary muscles resulting in abnormal cusp coaption and mitral regurgitation.

5. *Mitral annulus calcification*
   Primarily affects elderly females. Degenerative condition of the mitral annulus which may rarely spread to involve the conducting tissue. Frequently an incidental finding at post mortem, but there is a higher incidence in association with hypercalcaemia, diabetes mellitus and systemic hypertension. Calcification may act as a source of emboli or a focus for infection. Very rarely calcification is severe enough to cause inflow obstruction.

6. *Infective endocarditis*
   See Chapter 11.

7. *Hypertrophic cardiomyopathy*
   See Chapter 6.

8. *Connective tissue disease* (e.g. Marfan's syndrome, pseudoxanthoma elasticum, osteogenesis imperfecta)
   Rare. May be associated with regurgitation of other valves.

9. *Congenital defects* (mitral cleft, parachute valve)
   Very rare.

Pathophysiology

In chronic mitral regurgitation the resistance to left ventricular ejection is reduced and the left ventricular ejection time is shortened. Up to one third of the regurgitant fraction may be ejected into the left atrium prior to the opening of the aortic valve. The amount of mitral regurgitation is labile and depends on the size of the mitral orifice, the size of the left atrium, left atrial compliance, the size of the left ventricle and systemic vascular resistance. In acute mitral regurgitation there is a sudden rise in left atrial pressure with little change in left ventricular volume, whereas in chronic mitral regurgitation the left atrial compliance is low and the atrium dilates with little change in left atrial pressure. Late in the natural history of chronic mitral regurgitation the left ventricular end diastolic volume increases and this is a useful index of the likelihood of postoperative myocardial dysfunction.

Symptoms

1. *Asymptomatic*
   Patients may remain asymptomatic for many years with a gradual increase in mitral regurgitation and compensatory left ventricular dilatation and hypertrophy.

2. *Fatigue*
   Insidious onset of fatigue occurs when the regurgitant volume

exceeds the forward stroke volume and the effective cardiac output falls.

3. *Palpitations*

May take the form of an awareness of the hyperdynamic heartbeat, extrasystoles or episodes of sustained tachycardia, usually atrial fibrillation.

4. *Breathlessness*

Exertional breathlessness occurs late; symptoms of orthopnoea or nocturnal dyspnoea are uncommon.

5. *Other symptoms*

Symptoms related to systemic embolism or infective endocarditis can occur. Angina is rare in isolated mitral regurgitation.

Physical signs

1. *Pulse*

Normal pulse pressure. Sharp upstroke caused by premature aortic valve closure and a short ejection time.

2. *Venous pressure*

Normal unless there is pulmonary hypertension (prominent 'a' wave) or secondary tricuspid regurgitation (prominent systolic wave).

3. *Precordium*

Moderate or severe mitral regurgitation is associated with a displaced hyperdynamic apex beat often associated with a systolic thrill. The apical impulse becomes quieter with the development of ventricular impairment. A left parasternal impulse may be due to systolic expansion of the left atrium or right ventricular enlargement (uncommon).

4. *Heart sounds and murmurs*

S1 is normal or soft and S2 may be widely split due to premature aortic closure. An S3 accompanies mitral regurgitation of at least moderate severity. Mitral regurgitation due to a 'floppy' mitral valve may be associated with a click (or clicks) in the middle third of systole. An additional late systolic murmur indicates mild to moderate mitral regurgitation. As the regurgitation becomes more severe, the murmur lengthens and the click disappears. Typically, the murmur of mitral regurgitation is pansystolic commencing immediately after S1 and obscuring A2. The murmur is best heard at the apex radiating to the axilla, but if posterior chordal rupture has occurred the anteriorly directed jet may be heard at the left sternal edge and base radiating to the neck. The intensity of the murmur does not relate to the severity of the lesion.

Investigations

1. *Electrocardiography*
   Left atrial enlargement is reflected in the P mitrale. In mild
   to moderate mitral regurgitation the ECG may be normal,
   but with progression of the disease, evidence of left
   ventricular hypertrophy and 'strain' becomes apparent.
   Chronic atrial fibrillation develops in 75% of patients.

2. *Chest radiograph*
   In moderate to severe mitral regurgitation there is left
   ventricular dilatation causing an increase in the cardiothoracic
   ratio. Left atrial enlargement may reach aneurysmal
   proportions. Pulmonary venous congestion and interstitial
   pulmonary oedema occur late in the natural history of
   chronic mitral regurgitation.

3. *Echocardiography*
   Serial echocardiograms have largely replaced the chest
   radiograph in the follow-up of patients with chronic mitral
   regurgitation. In mild disease, left ventricular dimensions and
   systolic function are normal. In moderate regurgitation, the
   motion of the interventricular septum is hyperdynamic and
   the left ventricular filling rate during the first third of diastole
   is rapid. Later, the left ventricular and left atrial dimensions
   increase and systolic function deteriorates. The mitral valve
   appears non-rheumatic and may exhibit 'holosystolic' or late
   systolic prolapse of one or both leaflets. Chordal rupture,
   vegetations and flail leaflets can be identified on a
   cross-sectional study. Prominent systolic waves cause bowing of
   the interatrial septum towards the right side during ventricular
   systole.

   When ventricular disease is the primary diagnosis and
   mitral regurgitation is secondary, global impairment of
   systolic function is apparent on the cross-sectional study.
   Posterior wall movement is reduced, the interventricular
   septum is akinetic, end-diastolic dimension is increased and
   fractional shortening reduced. Mild to moderate concentric
   left ventricular hypertrophy occurs in longstanding mitral
   regurgitation.

4. *Doppler*
   Using a combination of continuous and pulsed wave Doppler
   a mitral regurgitant jet can be identified from the apical or
   parasternal position. Estimates can be made of the size, the
   direction and the velocity of the jet.

5. *Haemodynamics*
   In mild mitral regurgitation resting haemodynamics are
   normal, in particular the pulmonary artery capillary wedge

(PACW) pressure is low (>12 mmHg) but may increase on exercise. As the severity of the regurgitation increases, both the PACW pressure and the LVEDP increase. In a few patients PA and RA pressure are increased at rest. Prominent systolic waves are uncommon in long-standing mitral regurgitation.

6. *Cineangiography*

Cineangiography is performed using standard techniques (see Ch. 20). In mild disease the left ventricular dimensions and systolic function are normal. As the regurgitant fraction increases, LV dimensions increase and the active contraction pattern becomes less marked until eventually the ejection fraction falls. A semiquantitative estimate of the regurgitant fraction can be made from the degree of opacification of the left atrium although this is dependent both on left atrial size and left ventricular function.

Differential diagnosis

1. *Ventricular septal defect*

High pitched pansystolic murmur accompanied by a systolic thrill maximal at the left sternal edge. Pulmonary plethora may be apparent on the chest radiograph. Clinical differentiation between a post infarction ventricular septal defect and acute mitral regurgitation due to chordal or papillary muscle rupture may be impossible. The simplest method of confirming the diagnosis at the bed side is by detecting a step-up in oxygen saturation between RA and RV using a balloon directed (Swan-Ganz) flotation catheter (see Ch. 20).

2. *Tricuspid regurgitation*

Associated findings of fluid retention, an elevated venous pressure with prominent systolic waves and hepatic enlargement which may be pulsatile support a diagnosis of tricuspid regurgitation. The position and radiation of the murmur is unhelpful in distinguishing mitral from tricuspid regurgitation, but accentuation of the murmur in inspiration may occur in the latter.

3. *Aortic stenosis/sclerosis*

In the elderly patient, the ejection systolic murmur widely heard over the precordium must be differentiated from the pansystolic murmur of mitral regurgitation (e.g. from mitral annulus calcification). If there is significant left ventricular outflow obstruction, the carotid pulse will be modified, the lateral chest radiograph will show aortic valve calcification, and an echocardiogram will help to exclude aortic valve disease.

Natural history of chronic non-rheumatic mitral regurgitation

The natural history of non-rheumatic mitral regurgitation is very variable; some patients remain asymptomatic for many years, whereas in others there is rapid deterioration as a result of endocarditis, atrial fibrillation or rupture of further chordae. Prognosis is better than in patients with either mitral stenosis or mixed mitral valve disease with up to 80% of patients surviving 5 years and 60% living 10 years after diagnosis.

Medical management

1. *Diuretics*
   Moderate mitral regurgitation can usually be managed with small doses of diuretics.
2. *Digoxin*
   Ventricular rate is controlled with once daily digoxin in patients who are in established atrial fibrillation. If atrial fibrillation occurs in young patients (<50 years old) in whom the left atrium is not greatly enlarged, then DC cardioversion should be attempted and the use of quinidine should be considered (see Ch. 16).
3. *Arterial vasodilators*
   Recently, arterial vasodilators have been increasingly used for the patient with moderate mitral regurgitation, and some would advocate their use instead of diuretics (see Ch. 7).
4. *Anticoagulants*
   The place of anticoagulant therapy in chronic mitral regurgitation is controversial. Thromboembolism is less common than in mitral stenosis and anticoagulants should probably be reserved for patients with a history suggestive of emboli, those with intracardiac thrombus or giant left atrium on echocardiography, and patients with an unstable rhythm.

Indications for surgery

Patients with chronic mitral regurgitation should attend for regular follow-up every 6–12 months. Evidence of decreasing exercise tolerance (if necessary using formal exercise testing) or an increase in left ventricular dimensions determined by echocardiography are an indication for surgical intervention. The choice of procedure lies between mitral repair and replacement.

Mitral valve repair

If a surgeon is experienced in mitral reconstructive techniques, mitral repair is the procedure of choice for many types of non-rheumatic mitral regurgitation. Longterm results of repair of the posterior cusp are superior to procedures involving the anterior cusp or both cusps.

Numerous procedures have been devised including excision of redundant cusp tissue, chordal reimplantation and shortening and mitral annuloplasty with or without insertion of prosthetic ring. Early mortality is similar to mitral valve replacement, but the long-term complications of prosthetic valves are avoided, although a subgroup of patients will require reoperation for recurrence of mitral regurgitation.

Mitral valve replacement

If mitral repair is not possible or technically unsatisfactory then mitral valve replacement is undertaken. Choice of prosthesis and the results are similar to patients with mitral stenosis (see p. 147). A special subgroup are patients with ischaemic heart disease and mitral regurgitation who require mitral valve replacement concomitant coronary artery bypass grafting. The early mortality reflects the degree of myocardial dysfunction and may approach 15–20%, particularly if the procedure is carried out as an emergency.

Mitral valve prolapse syndrome

Isolated mitral valve prolapse can be regarded as a normal variant occurring in 5–15% of the population. In a proportion of patients this valve anomaly is associated with a more widespread spectrum of cardiac and extracardiac symptoms (Table 8.5).

Table 8. 5 Symptoms of mitral valve prolapse syndrome

1. Chest pain
2. Palpitations
3. Anxiety
4. Fatigue, lethargy and an inability to concentrate
5. Exercise intolerance
6. Postural symptoms

The syndrome is at present ill understood and there is a tendency for the physician to dismiss the symptoms as having no organic basis. It is important to take a careful history and examine the patient, confirming the presence of mitral valve prolapse by echocardiography. Evidence of pre-excitation or variable inferior repolarisation changes may be apparent on the resting ECG, and a 'false positive' exercise test is not uncommon. Arrhythmias, particularly atrial and ventricular premature beats are frequently documented on the resting ECG or by Holter monitoring. Sustained tachycardia (e.g. paroxysmal atrial tachycardia) is less common. Sudden death has been documented very rarely.

Once serious cardiac disease has been excluded, the mainstay of treatment is careful explanation and reassurance. Avoidance of stimulants (e.g. tea and coffee) may be helpful if arrhythmias are troublesome and in occasional patients a small dose of a beta blocker may beneficial (e.g. Atenolol 50 mg once daily). In general drugs are best avoided.

Investigation should usually stop short of invasive testing unless there is concern that there may be additonal coronary artery disease.

9. AORTIC VALVE DISEASE

AORTIC STENOSIS

Aetiology

1. *Congenital aortic stenosis*
   Congenital aortic stenosis occurs in 0.04% of live births, which represents 7% of all cases of congenital heart disease. In congenital aortic stenosis the valve resembles a dome with a central orifice, or alternatively has a single eccentric commisure with a slit-like opening.

2. *Acquired aortic stenosis*
   A number of forms of acquired aortic stenosis are seen in adult life including calcification of a tricuspid aortic valve, calcification of a congenitally bicuspid valve, rheumatic aortic stenosis, and mixed forms of aortic stenosis. Whereas only 40% of middle-aged patients with aortic stenosis have a bicuspid aortic valve, this type of aortic stenosis accounts for the majority (70–80%) of elderly patients. Rheumatic aortic stenosis in the absence of rheumatic mitral disease is uncommon accounting for only 2% of the total. Two points are worthy of note; firstly, a congenitally bicuspid valve (which occurs in approximately 2% of all live births) does not cause congenital aortic stenosis, but may lead to significant LV outflow obstruction in later life. Secondly, aortic valve calcification occurs in 5% of the population at autopsy and is *not* synonymous with aortic stenosis.

Pathophysiology

Aortic stenosis in the adult is a slowly progressive disease. Not until the aortic valve area is reduced from the normal 3 cm^2 to <1 cm^2 is there any significant haemodynamic derangement. In the face of an increasing outflow gradient, cardiac output is maintained by compensatory left ventricular hypertrophy at the expense of increased LV systolic wall stress and myocardial oxygen consumption. Early in the course of the disease cardiac output is normal at rest but fails to increase with exercise. Later, end diastolic volume increases, and the ventricle resembles that seen in dilated cardiomyopathy.

Emphasis in the early literature was related to the failure of the LV to eject (i.e. a primary abnormality of systolic function). More recent advances in the understanding of the pathophysiology of aortic stenosis include the appreciation of the importance of the derangement in diastolic function. Hypertrophy in this and other types of LV disease (e.g. hypertrophic cardiomyopathy) reduces LV compliance, inhibits normal ventricular filling, and compromises coronary blood flow.

Prolonged LV ejection also increases myocardial oxygen consumption, and shortens the period of coronary diastolic filling; the elevation in LV end diastolic pressure leads to a reduction in coronary perfusion pressure (aortic diastolic pressure — LVEDP), resulting in subendocardial ischaemia.

Symptoms

Most patients with aortic stenosis remain asymptomatic for many years, but once symptoms develop the prognosis is poor. Chest pain, breathlessness and syncope are the classic triad of symptoms in aortic stenosis.

1. *Chest pain*
   Chest pain typical of angina develops in 50–70% of patients with significant aortic stenosis. Whether chest pain is due to the aortic valve lesion or concomitant coronary artery disease (which is present in 10–50% of patients) cannot be differentiated on clinical grounds.

   Myocardial ischaemia results from a number of factors including increased myocardial oxygen demand (MVO_2) due to LV hypertrophy, prolonged ejection, increased wall stress, shortened coronary diastolic filling, and reduced coronary perfusion pressure. Rare causes of angina include coronary embolism or extension of the aortic valve calcification to involve the coronary ostia.

2. *Breathlessness*
   Reduced LV compliance and an elevated LV end diastolic pressure cause an increase in pulmonary venous pressure. Symptoms related to pulmonary venous hypertension occur late in the natural history of aortic valve stenosis and are associated with a poor prognosis. Initially, breathlessness occurs on exertion, but subsequently progressive dyspnoea, orthopnoea and nocturnal dyspnoea as a consequence of pulmonary oedema are present at rest.

3. *Dizziness and syncope*
   15–30% of symptomatic patients experience dizziness or syncope. During exertion, a fall in systemic vascular resistance (due to vasodilatation) in the patient with a fixed cardiac output causes a sudden reduction cerebral perfusion.

Less commonly, dizziness or syncope is caused by transient tachyarrhythmias, or atrioventricular block secondary to calcification extending from the aortic annulus into the interventricular septum and the conducting system. Sudden death has also been reported.

4. *Thromboembolism*
Transient ischaemic attacks or embolism to a major artery are unusual in aortic stenosis and are caused by calcium or platelet emboli arising from the valve or aortic root.
Transient blindness (amaurosis fugax) due to occlusion of the central retinal artery may also occur. In the elderly patient, cerebrovascular events are as likely to have arisen from the carotid bifurcation as from the aortic valve.

Physical signs

1. *Pulse*
The most important, and often neglected, physical sign in aortic stenosis is the character of the pulse. Examination of the carotid pulse reveals a slow upstroke as a result of prolonged ejection, and a small pulse pressure (pulsus parvus et tardus). A palpable (anacrotic) notch may be palpable on the upstroke, together with coarse systolic vibrations (carotid shudder). In the elderly, reduced elasticity of the peripheral arteries may mask the abnormalities in the pulse even when the lesion is severe. Additional aortic regurgitation may complicate the interpretation of the arterial waveform. In severe aortic stenosis pulsus alternans may be observed, but this also occurs in many other forms of LV disease.

2. *Venous pressure*
A prominent 'a' wave (Bernheim 'a' wave) can occasionally be seen in the venous pressure due to reduced RV distensibility secondary to hypertrophy of the interventricular septum.

3. *Precordial impulses*
A sustained apex beat is compatible with LV hypertrophy, and a pre-systolic 'a' wave may also be palpable. Only when LV dilatation has occurred in end-stage aortic stenosis, or if there is additional aortic regurgitation, is the apex beat displaced laterally. A systolic thrill, if present, is best appreciated with the flat of the hand applied to the precordium over the base of the heart with the patient leaning forward. The presence of a thrill is not related to the severity of the valve lesion.

4. *Heart sounds and murmurs*
S1 is normal or reduced. Calcification and rigidity of the aortic valve causes A2 to be diminished or inaudible, and

additional ventricular disease results in prolonged LV ejection. Both these mechanisms cause S2 to be single, narrowly split or paradoxical depending on the severity of the stenosis and the degree of LV dysfunction. Accentuation of P2 indicates that the aortic valve disease is complicated by pulmonary hypertension.

Elevation of the left atrial pressure results in an audible S4, which in young patients is indicative of severe outflow obstruction. Whilst the valve retains some mobility a high pitched systolic ejection click can be heard approximately 60 ms after S1. An ejection click is heard less frequently in adults, but in children the presence of an ejection click confirms that the obstruction is at valvar level.

A harsh systolic crescendo-decrescendo (ejection) murmur accompanies aortic stenosis. On auscultation, the murmur is maximal at the left sternal edge and radiates to the 'aortic area' and the carotid arteries. Neither the intensity, nor the length of the murmur is reliable in estimating the severity of the obstruction. Indeed, the elderly patient in pulmonary oedema with a low cardiac output may have little or no murmur (because of low forward flow) despite severe aortic stenosis.

Typically, the murmur starts after S1, and terminates prior to S2. This helps to differentiate between aortic stenosis and mild mitral regurgitation; in the latter, the murmur is longer and ends at S2. In non-rheumatic mitral regurgitation secondary to prolapse of the posterior mitral cusp the regurgitant jet is directed anteriorly and is audible at the base of the heart, in a similar area to the murmur of aortic stenosis. Degenerative changes of the aortic valve (aortic sclerosis) of no haemodynamic consequence may give rise to an ejection systolic murmur, but the key to determining the severity of the obstruction is a careful analysis of the carotid upstroke.

Investigations

1. *Electrocardiography*
   An abnormal ECG is seen in 70–80% of patients with aortic stenosis, but it is important to emphasize that a normal ECG does not exclude the presence of severe aortic stenosis. Correlation between ECG evidence of LV hypertrophy and LV mass determined at postmortem is poor. ECG features of LV hypertrophy are shown in Table 9.1. Minor repolarisation abnormalities (e.g. T wave inversion) are non-specific and unreliable. Although serial ECGs are more useful than a single recording in monitoring progress of disease,

Table 9.1 ECG features of left ventricular hypertrophy*

1. R wave (V_4, V_5) >27 mm
2. S Wave (V_1, V_2 or V_3) >30 mm
3. Tallest R wave + tallest S wave >40 mm
4. Ventricular activation time >40 ms
5. Anterolateral ST segment depression (>1 mm)
6. Anterolateral T wave inversion

*None of these findings are specific; the more criteria fulfilled, the more likely the diagnosis of LVH

echocardiography is a more sensitive method of assessing the severity of aortic stenosis and LV hypertrophy. Exercise stress testing has been used to follow children with aortic stenosis.

Evidence of left atrial hypertrophy (biphasic P wave in V1) is a frequent finding. First degree atrioventricular block, left axis deviation, LBBB or complete heart block indicate myocardial fibrosis, or extension of the calcium from the aortic annulus into the conducting system.

Atrial fibrillation is uncommon in uncomplicated aortic stenosis and may indicate concomitant mitral valve disease.

2. *Chest radiograph*

In uncomplicated aortic stenosis the cardiothoracic ratio is normal. Cardial enlargement indicates additional aortic regurgitation, mitral valve disease, or end-stage aortic stenosis with LV dilatation. Dilatation of the ascending aorta (post-stenotic dilatation) is present in 80% of patients but may be difficult to appreciate in the elderly because of aortic ectasia. In young patients the absence of post-stenotic dilatation suggests that the LV outflow tract obstruction is not at valve level.

The hallmark of aortic stenosis is aortic valve calcification. In the patient over 35 years of age the absence of calcification excludes significant aortic stenosis at valve level. The converse is not true; aortic valve calcification is a common finding in elderly patients, and need not indicate a significant aortic gradient. Calcification is best appreciated on the lateral chest radiograph; indeed, the PA film may appear entirely normal because calcium is difficult to visualise in this projection. Fluoroscopy aids in the identification of aortic valve calcification.

Aortic valve calcification may be the only clue to the aetiology of acute pulmonary oedema in a previously fit patient, therefore careful inspection of a lateral chest radiograph in these patients is mandatory.

3. *M-mode and cross-sectional echocardiography*

Abnormalities of the aortic valve can be readily identified by echocardiography although the presence and severity of aortic stenosis is less easy to determine. Eccentricity of the aortic closure line does not reliably identify a bicuspid valve and thickening of the aortic cusps and restriction of leaflet motion visualised by M-mode echocardiography may merely indicate aortic valve calcification or an off axis recording. Congenital aortic stenosis is particularly difficult to assess because leaflet motion may appear normal at the level of the aortic annulus despite restriction of the effective orifice at the apex of the valve. Cross-sectional echocardiography is more reliable in detecting leaflet motion and coaption of the cusps, and can differentiate between valvar aortic stenosis and other forms of left ventricular outflow obstruction. By either technique, LV hypertrophy can be demonstrated often in association with a small ventricular cavity. Assessment of LV function frequently gives as much information as the examination of the valve itself. Non-invasive estimates of the LV outflow gradient derived from the severity of LV hypertrophy are unreliable as they presuppose normal LV function.

4. *Doppler*

Maximal systolic pressure difference across the aortic valve can be detected by Doppler using the maximal velocity value. Limitations of this technique are similar to haemodynamic measurements in that estimates of the gradient are unreliable in patients with a low cardiac output. More recently, Doppler has also been used to estimate cardiac output, and if this application is found to be reliable, the technique will be invaluable in the assessment of the patient with aortic stenosis.

5. *Cardiac catheterisation*

LV function and the outflow gradient can be determined by cardiac catheterisation using standard techniques. Difficulty may be encountered in crossing a stenotic valve, particularly when the lesion is severe. Prolonged attempts at crossing a diseased aortic valve may be poorly tolerated as the catheter itself can significantly obstruct the available lumen. Alternative approaches include direct LV puncture and transseptal catheterisation to obtain the pressure within the LV body which is then compared with a simultaneously recorded aortic pressure. Aortic valve area can be calculated from the Gorlin formula. Angiographic evidence of LV hypertrophy includes prominence of the papillary muscles, reduced LV dimensions and cavity obliteration at end systole. The stenotic valve appears thickened and irregular with reduced cusp mobility and a small orifice.

Most cardiac surgeons will require delineation of the coronary artery anatomy before proceeding to aortic valve replacement in order to determine the need for concomitant coronary artery bypass grafting. As the need for aortic valve replacement is usually clear on clinical grounds, an aortogram and coronary arteriograms are sufficient if there is difficulty in crossing the aortic valve in which case LV function can be determined by echocardiography.

Other types of left ventricular outflow obstruction

1. *Discrete subaortic stenosis*

   Discrete subaortic stenosis accounts for 20% of left ventricular outflow tract obstruction in infants and young children. Symptoms are similar to those of aortic stenosis. On examination an ejection systolic murmur is audible, which is indistinguishable from that of valvar aortic stenosis. Changes in S2 are variable. Patients with subaortic stenosis do not have an ejection click, and the absence of a click in a child strongly suggests that the outflow obstruction is not at valve level. The aortic valve in patients with aortic stenosis is usually tricuspid, but may be thickened and mildly regurgitant due to the 'jet' impinging on the valve leaflets. Hence, these patients are liable to infective endocarditis.

   LV hypertrophy is evident on the ECG, but the chest radiograph is frequently unremarkable. Unlike the patient with valvar stenosis, post stenotic dilatation of the aorta is absent. Echocardiography reveals a discrete membrane, crescentic in shape, just below the aortic valve. Premature closure of the aortic valve on M-mode echocardiography is not specific for this condition, but it is a useful finding because it is not a feature of other causes of discrete LV outflow obstruction. Cardiac catheterisation reveals a subaortic chamber, with a subvalve gradient. Cineangiography is best carried out using angled views to profile the outflow tract (Ch. 20). An aortogram may demonstrate mild aortic regurgitation.

   Resection of the membrane and complete relief of the obstruction can be accomplished at low risk with excellent symptomatic and functional improvement.

2. *Tunnel subaortic stenosis*

   This rare condition is frequently associated with other cardiac anomalies (e.g. small aortic annulus, hypoplastic ascending aorta, coarctation of the aorta). Physical findings are similar to discrete subaortic stenosis, and the narrowed outflow tract can be identified by echocardiography. Unlike discrete subaortic stenosis, operative intervention has a significant risk with variable results.

3. *Hypertrophic obstructive cardiomyopathy*

   See Chapter 6.

4. *Supravalvar aortic stenosis*

   Supravalvar aortic stenosis is the least common type of LV

outflow obstruction. A number of varieties have been described of which a discrete waist-like narrowing of the ascending aorta is the most common. Autosomal dominant inheritance has been described, and other children have associated hypercalcaemia, mental retardation, and characteristic (elfin) facies. Sudden death in this condition is not infrequent.

Physical findings are typical of LV outflow tract obstruction with no ejection click. Differences in the character of the carotid pulses has been attributed to the Bernoulli effect. Surgical correction is feasible, but the outcome is dependent on the associated lesions.

Medical management

There is little place for medical management in the patient with significant aortic valve stenosis. Once symptoms develop most patients die within three years. Aortic stenosis is a mechanical problem, and is not responsive to diuretics or vasodilators. Over diuresis may actually exacerbate the haemodynamics by depleting intravascular volume and reducing 'preload'. Prophylaxis against infective endocarditis in situations of potential infection is an important precaution (Ch. 11).

Surgery

Symptoms attributable to aortic stenosis warrant surgical intervention. Because the aortic gradient is dependent on cardiac output, an absolute value does not determine whether surgical intervention is or is not appropriate; however, most patients who require surgery have a peak systolic gradient of at least 50 mmHg. Expected early mortality from aortic valve replacement is 5–10%. Determinants of increased operative risk include preoperative pulmonary hypertension, and additional mitral valve disease or coronary artery disease. Increasing chronological age is not a contraindication to aortic valve replacement. Aortic valve replacement should be contemplated in any patient with aortic stenosis, even if LV function is severely compromised. Despite the increased risk of surgery some of these patients do surprisingly well.

The choice of prosthesis depends on the age of the patient and the preference of the surgeon. Although there is considerable variation in the haemodynamic profiles of the various types of valve available, symptomatic benefit is similar and patient-valve mismatch is uncommon. Ball and cage valves (e.g. Starr-Edwards 1260) are not suited to patients with a small aortic root and annulus, as the effective orifice area is less than half that of valves with a central opening (e.g. St Jude). Doubts concerning the durability of tissue valves (e.g. Carpentier-Edwards porcine xenograft), are less important in elderly patients, and they have the added advantage that they do not require formal anticoagulation which may be hazardous in this age group. Similarly, young female patients who are considering pregnancy may be well advised to consider a tissue valve because of the difficulties in managing anticoagulants in pregnancy. In other young adults a mechanical valve is preferable.

Infants presenting with congenital aortic stenosis in the first year of life can be regarded as a separate group and do poorly due to severe LV disease and a valve that does not lend itself to a conservative procedure. Operative mortality in infants is 20–40%. In children and young adults, open aortic valvotomy is an excellent palliative operation with an early mortality of <3%. Despite the possibility of a small residual gradient or surgically induced aortic regurgitation, these are usually well tolerated and allow the child (and the aortic annulus) to grow for 10–15 years until a prosthesis can be inserted. Thus, the complications of managing anticoagulants in children, or the risks of premature calcification in a tissue valve are avoided.

Various series predict a five year survival of 70–88%, and a 10 year survival of 60–73% following aortic valve replacement. Thromboembolic rates vary from 6.5 per 100 patient-years of follow-up for Starr-Edwards valves to <1 thromboembolic events per 100 patient-years for the Carpentier-Edwards xenograft. In situ thrombosis has been reported in 2% of tilting disc valves (e.g. Bjork-Shiley). In mechanical valves, 10% of patients experience complications from oral anticoagulants (warfarin), and 1% of patients die from these complications. Valve dysfunction in tissue valves can be detected in up to 5% of patients at five years, and 5–12% of patients at eight years.

AORTIC REGURGITATION

Aetiology

Chronic aortic regurgitation may be due to disease of the aortic valve or the aortic root (Table 9.2). Degenerative and connective tissue diseases of the aortic root cause dilatation of the annulus and the ascending aorta, but as the aortic valve itself may be normal it can frequently be conserved when abnormality of the root is corrected by surgery.

Acute aortic regurgitation may result from infective endocarditis, aortic dissection or trauma. Infective endocarditis causes aortic regurgitation by destruction or perforation of a leaflet usually in a previously bicuspid valve. Retrograde extension of a dissecting haematoma as a cause of acute aortic regurgitation is discussed in Chapter 10. Acute aortic regurgitation is the valve lesion most commonly encountered in patients with closed chest trauma (e.g. steering wheel compression injuries). Isolated spontaneous rupture or prolapse of an aortic cusp has also been described and may represent a forme fruste of the Marfan syndrome.

Table 9.2 Aetiology of chronic aortic regurgitation

1. Cusp abnormality:	Perforation	Infective endocarditis
	Reduction in area	Rheumatic disease Rheumatoid Ankylosing spondylitis
2. Aortic root disease:	Root distortion	Rheumatoid Ankylosing spondylitis Syphilis Non-specific urethritis Non-specific aortitis
	Root dilatation	Syphilis Marfan's syndrome Ehlers-Danlos syndrome Pseudoxanthoma elasticum Other types of aortitis

Pathophysiology

Severity of aortic regurgitation is determined by the aortic valve area, the heart rate (particularly the length of diastole), and the diastolic pressure gradient between the LV and the aorta. Thus, the regurgitant fraction can be altered by changes in systemic vascular resistance (afterload) and adversely affected by bradycardia.

Chronic aortic regurgitation results in diastolic overload and LV dilatation. In the dilated heart systolic wall stress is maintained by compensatory LV hypertrophy. Eventually, LV end diastolic volume increases still further in association with a fall in cardiac output and pulmonary venous hypertension.

The abrupt onset of acute aortic regurgitation allows no time for dilatation and hypertrophy to develop; a sudden increase in LVEDP with little change in LV end diastolic volume precipitates acute pulmonary oedema.

Symptoms

Aortic regurgitation is well tolerated. Most patients remain asymptomatic until late in the disease, by which time considerable LV dysfunction has occurred. Restriction of exercise tolerance due to breathlessness and fatigue are followed by symptoms of pulmonary oedema and fluid retention. Angina pectoris is less common than in aortic stenosis, but a syndrome of nocturnal angina associated with profuse sweating in young patients with severe aortic regurgitation and normal coronary arteries has been described. Pain without the features of cardiac ischaemia may arise from the aortic root. Syncope is rare. Palpitations, taking the form of an awareness of the heart beat due to the increased stroke volume and wide pulse pressure, are particularly noticeable whilst lying down at rest.

Physical signs

The general appearance of the patient may give a clue to the nature of
the aortic valve disease. Features of connective tissue disease (e.g.
Marfan's syndrome, Ehlers-Danlos syndrome), or joint disorders (e.g.
rheumatoid arthritis, ankylosing spondylitis) may be immediately
apparent. A careful search for the stigmata of infective endocarditis is
important in patients with acute aortic regurgitation.

1. *Pulse*

   The striking findings in aortic regurgitation relate to the wide
   pulse pressure and rapid diastolic runoff. Palpation of the
   carotid reveals a full volume pulse of short duration with a
   sharp upstroke. A carotid systolic thrill or shudder on the upstroke may be present in pure aortic regurgitation. A number
   of eponymous signs from the older literature are still used to
   describe various features of the wide pulse pressure (e.g.
   Quincke's and Duroziez's signs). A sphygmomanometer
   recording of the blood pressure may indicate a pulse pressure
   exceeding 100 mmHg, but the detection of the Korotkoff 4th
   (muffling) or 5th (disappearance) phases in these
   circumstances may be impossible.

2. *Venous pressure*

   Prominent arterial pulsations in the neck may make
   interpretation of the venous waveform difficult. True
   elevation in the venous pressure is not apparent until late in
   the disease.

3. *Precordial impulses*

   An active hyperdynamic apex beat of short duration is
   present, which is displaced inferiorly and laterally due to LV
   dilatation. A rapid filling wave may also be palpable in early
   diastole together with a systolic thrill.

4. *Heart sounds and murmurs*

   S1 is normal, or may be soft in first degree atrioventricular
   block. In acute aortic regurgitation S1 is quiet because of
   premature mitral closure (see p. 168). S2 is variable
   depending on the mobility of the valve. An S4 may be
   audible due to the left atrium contracting into a non-
   compliant ventricle, and an S3 either indicates rapid filling or
   LV dilatation. A systolic ejection click if present relates to
   sudden distension of the aortic root.

   A high pitched soft early diastolic murmur starting
   immediately after A2 is the typical feature of aortic
   regurgitation. It is best heard with the diaphragm of the
   stethoscope applied quite firmly to the precordium over the
   left sternal edge. The patient is asked to lean forward, exhale
   and then to stop breathing, and the stethoscope is moved up
   and down the left sternal edge because the murmur may be

well localised in position and of short duration especially if the lesion is mild. Severity of the regurgitation is related to the length not the loudness of the murmur. In aortic cusp prolapse or perforation, the murmur may be high pitched with a musical quality (seagull or cooing dove murmur).

Increased stoke volume creates a systolic flow murmur, similar in character to the murmur of aortic stenosis. Moderate to severe aortic regurgitation is accompanied by a low pitched, mid diastolic rumbling murmur identical in character and location to that of mitral stenosis (Austin Flint murmur). Theories of the causation of this murmur in the absence of organic mitral valve disease include a mitral flow murmur secondary to rapid forward flow, or functional mitral stenosis caused by oscillation of the anterior mitral leaflet by the regurgitant jet. Organic mitral disease can be differentiated on clinical grounds by the quiet S1, absent opening snap, and the fact that patients with isolated aortic valve disease are usually in sinus rhythm.

In acute aortic regurgitation the physical signs are frequently unimpressive leading to an under estimation of the severity of the lesion. The patient appears unwell with breathlessness at rest and a tachycardia, but the signs relating to the wide pulse pressure are absent and in the presence of pulmonary oedema the murmurs may be inaudible. Pulsus alternans and a loud S3 are clues to the severity of the lesion.

Investigations

1. *Electrocardiography*
   In chronic aortic regurgitation the ECG is rarely normal. Features of LV hypertrophy are present (see p. 160) with increased precordial voltages, poor anterior R wave progression and repolarisation abnormalities. A biphasic P wave in V1 is indicative of an elevated left atrial pressure. First degree atrioventricular block suggests disease of the aortic root, and left axis deviation and LBBB occur with progressive LV disease. In acute aortic regurgitation the ECG may be entirely normal.

2. *Chest radiograph*
   Chronic aortic regurgitation causes progressive cardiac enlargement due to dilatation of the LV. On the chest radiograph the heart enlarges in the transverse diameter. Diseases affecting the aortic root cause enlargement of the ascending aorta which may become aneurysmal. Aortic valve calcification is uncommon in pure aortic regurgitation. In acute aortic regurgitation, a normal heart size in association

with the radiographic features of acute pulmonary oedema is typical.

3. *M-mode and cross-sectional echocardiography*

Increased LV cavity dimensions, an active pattern of contraction and rapid filling are typical of chronic aortic regurgitation. With long-standing regurgitation LV systolic function becomes depressed and the ventricle may resemble that of dilated cardiomyopathy. Concentric LV hypertrophy is less impressive than in patients with aortic stenosis. Serial assessment of LV function by echocardiography allows decisions to be made with regard to the optimal timing of surgery.

Aortic regurgitation causes high frequency diastolic fluttering of the anterior leaflet of the mitral valve and less commonly fluttering of the interventricular septum. Organic mitral valve disease can be reliably excluded by the appearance of a normal mitral valve. Dilatation of the ascending aorta in association with a normal tricuspid aortic valve confirms disease of the aorta root. In Marfan's syndrome the aortic root has a typical flask-shaped appearance, and in aorta dissection a false lumen may be visualised.

In acute aortic regurgitation, severe regurgitation into an LV of normal size and low compliance results in premature closure of the mitral valve (i.e. elevated LV end diastolic pressure causes the mitral valve to close prior to the QRS complex). Premature mitral closure is an indication for urgent aortic valve replacement. Aortic vegetations, aortic leaflet prolapse, cusp perforation and abscesses in the interventricular septum complicating endocarditis may be visualised by echocardiography.

4. *Doppler*

Sensitivity and specificity of Doppler in the detection of aortic regurgitation exceeds 90%. A high frequency regurgitant jet can be detected in the outflow tract, and mapping of the jet with simultaneous cross-sectional echocardiography can be used to determine the severity of the regurgitation.

5. *Radionuclide studies*

LV function may be assessed using gated blood pool scanning. Regurgitant fraction and the ratio of RV to LV stroke volume allow non-invasive estimation of the severity of the aortic regurgitation. A failure to increase ejection fraction with exercise may be an early indicator of LV dysfunction in aortic regurgitation.

6. *Cardiac catheterisation*

In mild-moderate aortic regurgitation the haemodynamics at rest may be entirely normal. As the disease progresses, there is evidence of impaired diastolic function, and reduced contractility. LV end diastolic pressure increases, as does PACWP. Eventually, chronic pulmonary hypertension leads to elevated right-sided pressures.

LV cineangiography in the right anterior oblique projection reveals a hyperdynamic ventricle which becomes dilated and hypocontractile with chronic regurgitation. A semiquantitative estimate of aortic regurgitation can be made by aortography. Contrast is injected rapidly (20–40 ml/s) into the ascending aorta 3 cms above the aortic valve, and the amount of contrast flowing back into the LV is graded 1–4. If the injection is made too close to the aortic valve, spurious aortic regurgitation may result from interference with normal valve function. Aortography in the left anterior oblique projection allows assessment of the aortic root (see Ch. 20).

Medical management

Prognosis in chronic aortic regurgitation is favourable with a 10 year survival of 50%. Mild asymptomatic aortic regurgitation needs no specific treatment other than prophylaxis against infective endocarditis. Patients with severe aortic regurgitation require aortic valve replacement. Management of the group with moderate aortic regurgitation and few if any symptoms present the most difficulty. Justification for delaying surgical intervention in these patients is the good prognosis and the likelihood of them surviving a number of years without a reduction in exercise tolerance. With time the development of LV dysfunction causes an increase in operative risk, with the possibility of a less satisfactory result due to persisting LV disease following surgery.

There is little place for medical treatment in chronic symptomatic aortic regurgitation. Although diuretics and arterial vasodilators have been advocated, it is probable that in the patient with symptoms surgery is more appropriate.

Acute aortic regurgitation is usually due to infective endocarditis and requires prompt surgical intervention (Ch. 11). Prolonged attempts at correcting acute pulmonary oedema with diuretics and vasodilators cannot be recommended. Delay increases the operative mortality and the chance of multisystem failure and there is little evidence to indicate that an incomplete course of antibiotics prior to aortic valve replacement increases the chance of prosthetic endocarditis.

Indications for surgery

Chronic aortic regurgitation
1. Symptomatic chronic aortic regurgitation.
2. Asymptomatic aortic regurgitation with evidence of increasing LV dimensions, or reduced systolic function on serial echocardiographic testing.

3. Asymptomatic patient with increasing LV voltage on serial ECGs.
4. Asymptomatic patient with a failure to increase ejection fraction on exercise using radionuclide studies.
5. Evidence of increasing dilatation of the ascending aorta (or aneurysm formation) demonstrated by chest radiography, echocardiography or thoracic CT.

Acute aortic regurgitation

1. Aortic regurgitation due to infective endocarditis.
2. Traumatic aortic regurgitation (e.g. laceration, compression injury).
3. Type I (Stanford Type A) aortic dissection.
4. Aortic cusp rupture or prolapse ('spontaneous' aortic regurgitation).

Surgery

Most patients undergoing surgery for aortic regurgitation will require aortic valve replacement. An aortic valvuloplasty may be technically feasible in some young patients who have prolapse of an aortic valve cusp.

Decisions regarding choice of prosthesis have been discussed in the section on aortic stenosis (see p. 163). Dilatation of the aortic root allows insertion of a large aortic prosthesis without difficulty. Early mortality for simple aortic valve replacement is approximately 5%. Although cardiac enlargement and impared LV function reduce the chance of a good symptomatic result, current methods of myocardial protection mean that most patients survive the procedure. Following operation, the mortality in the patient with poor LV function is 5% per annum.

For the patient with aortic regurgitation and a dilated ascending aortic one of a number of more major procedures may be required. A composite aortic valve-low porosity Dacron conduit with reimplantation of the coronary arteries is favoured for patients with Marfan's syndrome. Alternatively, resection and replacement of the ascending aorta down to the annulus may allow the aortic valve to be conserved.

10. AORTIC DISSECTION

An aortic dissection is caused by a haematoma in the middle to outer third of the aortic media which is associated with an intimal tear in more than 95% of cases.

Dissection of the aorta occurs in 5–10 patients/million population/year, which represents approximately 600 cases in the UK per annum. The autopsy incidence varies between one in 350 and 500 cases, but the diagnosis during life is commonly missed. With the advent of greater clinical awareness, and the more widespread application of newer non-invasive techniques, the recognition and appropriate management of this frequently lethal condition should be possible.

AETIOLOGY

Pathogenesis of aortic dissection in the majority of cases relates to:
1. *Systemic hypertension*
   A factor in 75–90% of patients, dissection occurring in 0.5–1.0% of patients with significant elevation of BP.
2. *Connective tissue degeneration*
   Frequently a combination of an elastic tissue lesion (cystic medionecrosis), and smooth muscle lesion (laminar necrosis).
3. *The intimal tear*
   Flexing stress on the ascending (and descending) aorta caused by the arch being 'fixed' relative to the remainder of the aorta.
4. *Propagation of the dissecting haematoma*
   Related to dp/dt_{max} and the systemic blood pressure.

Less common conditions associated with aortic dissection are detailed in Table 10.1.

Table 10.1 Conditions associated with aortic dissection

1. Pregnancy
   Wide pulse pressure, increased heart rate and cardiac output, hormonal effects on connective tissues
2. Coarctation of the aorta
   If left untreated, 20% of these patients die from aortic dissection and/or rupture
3. Aortic stenosis
   Rare. Post stenotic dilatation from turbulent flow (the 'jet' lesion)
4. Turner's syndrome
   High incidence of elevated BP and/or coarctation
5. Marfan's syndrome
   Dissections occur particularly in pregnancy (50% in the third trimester)
6. Ehlers-Danlos syndrome (type III collagen deficiency)
   Rare
7. Giant cell arteritis
   Rare
8. Syphilis
   Rare
9. Relapsing polychondritis
   Rare
10. Familial dissection
    ? exists when Marfan's and Ehlers-Danlos syndromes excluded
11. Arteriosclerosis
    Intimal tears rarely occur through atheromatous plaques (2–4%)
12. Trauma
    Rare, e.g.steering wheel compression injury
13. Iatrogenic
    Inadvertent intramural injection of contrast medium during cardiac catheterisation

CLASSIFICATION

Definitions are based on the site of the intimal tear and the extent of the dissection. The DeBakey (1965) and Stanford (1970) classifications are in common use (Fig. 10.1).

DeBakey	Site	Stanford
Type I	Extends beyond ascending aorta	Type A
Type II	Confined to ascending aorta	Type A
Type III	Distal to L. subclavian artery	Type B

Anatomical sites of tears and rupture

60% of primary (or entry) tears are in the ascending aorta of which 50% are within 2 cm of the aortic valve. Tears become less frequent as the distance from the aortic ring increases. This distribution is almost certainly a function of the Laplace equation which relates circumferential wall tension to vessel diameter (which is greater in the ascending aorta) as well as intravascular pressure. Secondary (or re-entry) tears, usually in the iliac vessels or abdominal aorta, are encountered in only 15% of patients but are associated with a more favourable prognosis.

Dissection of the aorta tends to propagate distally rather than proximally giving rise to characteristic symptom complexes as major branches are compressed or occluded.

De Bakey classification

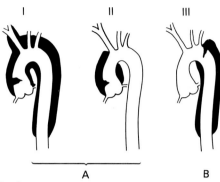

Stanford classification

Fig. 10.1 Classification of aortic dissection

The site of aortic rupture is related to the site of the primary tear, in dissections of the ascending aorta, 70% rupture into the pericardium, 6% into the left pleura and 6% into the mediastinum. Rarely, an aorta with a double lumen may develop in a patient who survives an acute dissection, the so-called 'healed' dissection.

SYMPTOMS

Symptoms of aortic dissection are commonly related to the site of the intimal tear. Although the incidence of dissection favours a proximal rather than a distal site (4:1), distal dissections come to medical attention more frequently as the prognosis of these lesions is more benign. Overall, 75% of patients are aged 40–70 years, and males are affected more commonly than females (2–3:1). Negroes are affected more frequently than Caucasians (probably due to the increased incidence of hypertension) and the finding of aortic dissection in Orientals is rare.

Acute symptoms

1. *Pain (90%)*
   Typically an excruciating, tearing or ripping sensation starting in the retrosternal region, and radiating to the dorsal spine (particularly in patients with distal dissection), the neck, jaw, throat etc. Pain tends to migrate with progression of the haematoma, and unlike the pain of acute myocardial ischaemia is maximal at its onset. Many patients experience additional vasovagal symptoms.

2. *Syncope (5–10%)*
   Usually from low cardiac output secondary to pericardial tamponade.
3. *Breathlessness (4–7%)*
   As a result of acute aortic regurgitation caused by disruption of the aortic valve ring.
4. *Cerebrovascular accident (2–3%)*
5. *Limb ischaemia*
6. *Anuria*
   Involvement of one or both renal arteries can result in renal impairment.
7. *Asymptomatic (2%)*

Chronic symptoms

Present with progressive effort dyspnoea as result of aortic regurgitation. Pain is either absent or prior pain was misdiagnosed.

PHYSICAL SIGNS

1. *Shock (25%)*
   In the majority of patients 'shock' is associated with an elevated blood pressure (evidence of pre-existing hypertension). In 20% of proximal dissections the BP is low due to pericardial tamponade or blood loss.
   NB: Pseudohypotension may occur as a result of involvement of the right brachial artery in the dissection.
2. *Lost or delayed pulse*
   May be transient due to flap movement or re-entry. Any pulse can be lost, but the finding is more common with a proximal dissection.
3. *Aortic regurgitation*
   Mechanisms involved in the development of aortic regurgitation include widening of the aortic root by a circumferential haematoma, displacement of one aortic cusp inferiorly or a flail aortic cusp secondary to disruption of the annulus. 30–60% of patients with a proximal dissection have aortic regurgitation, compared with <10% of those with a distal dissection. Typical signs of aortic regurgitation may be masked by a low cardiac output.
4. *Acute pulmonary oedema*
   Respiratory crackles are present in 10% of cases, and signs compatible with a pleural effusion (haemothorax) in 6%.
5. *Pericardial effusion (5–10%)*
   Clinical signs of pericardial tamponade may be associated

with rapid clinical deterioration. In contrast to acute myocardial infarction, a friction rub is uncommon.

6. *Neurological deficit*

    Altered consciousness occurs in up to 20% of patients, particularly in those with a proximal dissection, whereas in the distal group ischaemic neuropathy of the lower limbs is not infrequent. Other signs include a hemiparesis (3%), monoparesis (6%), and a paraparesis caused by spinal ischaemia (5%). Only 2% of patients experience visual disturbance. Horner's syndrome due to superior cervical ganglion involvement, and hoarseness of the voice from recurrent laryngeal nerve compression are both rare.

7. *Other physical signs*

    Numerous other less common signs have been reported in association with an aortic dissection including a pulsatile neck mass, superior vena caval obstruction, tracheo bronchial compression, haematemesis, acute myocardial, mesenteric or renal infarction, and rupture into the right atrium or ventricle. Finally, a dissection is a rare cause of an unexplained fever.

DIFFERENTIAL DIAGNOSIS

Thoracic: Acute myocardial infarction
Abdominal: Acute pancreatitis
    Mesenteric arterial or venous thrombosis
    Peptic ulceration
    Gastric carcinoma
    Pancreatic cyst
    Acute cholecystitis
    Appendicitis

INVESTIGATIONS

1. Mild anaemia from blood loss
2. Leukocytosis (10–14 000)
3. Disseminated intravascular coagulation (rare)
4. Haemolysis ($\uparrow$ LDH, $\uparrow$ bilirubin)
5. SGOT, CPK normal (vs acute myocardial infarction)
6. Electrocardiography. May be compatible with left ventricular hypertrophy

RADIOLOGY

1. *Chest radiograph*

   Abnormalities include widening of the superior mediastinum, a disparity in size between ascending and descending aorta, a double aortic shadow, radiolucency of the false lumen, an irregular aortic contour, loss of sharpness of the aorta and displaced intimal calcification. The cardiothoracic ratio can be increased due to pre-existing systemic hypertension, aortic regurgitation or a pericardial effusion. Signs of pulmonary oedema may be apparent. In 5–20% of patients the routine PA and left lateral chest radiograph is normal.

   Signs suggesting aortic dissection on the plain chest radiograph are non-specific, particularly if the film is portable (AP) and supine. Specificity is increased if sequential films are available for comparison.

2. *Aortography*

   The diagnosis of aortic dissection can be made with certainty by aortography in 90–99% of patients. An aortogram will define the extent of the dissection, the site of entry and re-entry, the involvement of major branches (including the coronary arteries), and allow assessment of the severity of aortic regurgitation. There is debate as to whether the femoral or brachial approach is preferable. Most advocate a percutaneous femoral approach using the Seldinger technique. In general a peripheral artery is chosen in which there is a strong pulse. A 7F or 8F pigtail catheter is cautiously advanced retrogradely until the tip is 3–5 cm from the aortic annulus. Once the catheter has entered the artery the guide wire should be removed as it may become caught under an intimal flap as the catheter is advanced. Great care is taken to monitor the arterial pressure through the catheter during the procedure as a damped pressure suggests that the catheter is lying within the false lumen. If this is the case, the catheter is withdrawn a few cms, and a small hand contrast injection (2–4 ml) is given to confirm the anatomy. Not uncommonly the catheter will pass from the true lumen to the false lumen and back without difficulty. Either cut film using a rapid film changer, or cineangiography may be used. A single plane left anterior oblique or anteroposterior projection is adequate. Once the catheter is positioned correctly, a pressure injection of 40–50 ml of Conray (or similar contrast agent) is injected at 20 ml/s. If cineangiography is used, the camera is panned from the aortic root to the bifurcation. A second injection at the level of the arch or descending aorta may be necessary to clearly visualise the distal thoracic and abdominal aorta and point of re-entry.

Signs of aortic dissection include an intimal flap, a double lumen, a compressed true lumen, a thickened aortic wall, lack of opacification of a major branch and aortic regurgitation. Absence of the left or right nephrogram suggests involvement of one or other renal artery in the dissection.

Even in critically ill patients the procedure is usually well tolerated, and the incidence of major complications is <1%.

COMPUTED TOMOGRAPHY

Computed tomography (CT) is an invaluable non-invasive diagnostic technique in the recognition and evaluation of the patient with an aortic dissection. Using contrast enhancement, an aortic dissection can be demonstrated in the majority of patients and the differentiation of an aortic dissection from an aortic aneurysm is possible. A number of CT criteria of dissection have been formulated of which detection of an intimal flap is the most specific.

CT findings in aortic dissection:
1. Detection of an intimal flap
2. Identification of two lumina
3. Displaced intimal calcification from outer aortic contour
4. Aortic lumen widening
5. Associated complications (e.g. pleural effusion, haemopericardium)

At present CT is used in conjunction with aortography, rather than obviating the need for invasive radiology. Sequential CT studies in medically treated patients have shown thrombosis of the false lumen or extension of the haematoma, thus aiding in the decision of whether to pursue conservative management.

Digital vascular imaging (DVI) offers promise in the investigation of aortic dissection, with the possibility of selective imaging of the true and false lumen and the analysis of differential flow characteristics within each channel.

ECHOCARDIOGRAPHY

Ultrasound complements CT in the investigation of aortic dissection. The regions of the aorta accessible to the M-mode beam are limited, but using the cross sectional technique with multiple non-conventional views virtually the whole length of the aorta can be imaged. The superior repetition rate of M-mode echocardiography should be utilised whenever possible (e.g. in imaging the ascending aorta), in conjunction with the cross sectional technique when necessary. Furthermore, echocardiography can be used to assess the severity of aortic regurgitation, associated left ventricular dysfunction and the presence or absence of a pericardial effusion.

Echocardiographic features of aortic dissection:

1. Recognition of intimal flaps oscillating within the aorta
2. Aortic root dilatation
3. Widening of aortic walls
4. Maintenance of parallel motion of aortic root walls
5. Preservation of aortic leaflet motion
6. Associated complications
   a. Aortic regurgitation: Diastolic fluttering of mitral valve and interventricular septum, rapid ventricular filling, LV dilatation, premature mitral closure
   b. Pericardial effusion or tamponade
   c. Left pleural effusion

TREATMENT OF AORTIC DISSECTION

The ideal management of the patient with an aortic dissection requires an integrated approach between medical and surgical therapy utilising the combination of investigative techniques described previously. Aortic dissection is a lethal condition, but studies of the natural history of untreated dissection reveal that only 3% of patients die immediately, 21% die within 24 hours, 60% within two weeks and 90% within 3 months. In the majority of patients there is time to plan appropriate investigation and treatment.

Initial management in all patients with suspected acute aortic dissection

1. Transfer to intensive care unit
2. Insert large bore (16 or 18G) central venous line
3. Insert arterial catheter into limb with palpable pulse
4. Insert urinary catheter and measure output hourly
5. Routine haematology and clotting profile, biochemistry, group and save serum
6. PA chest radiograph (standing or sitting)
7. Electrocardiogram (12 lead), and continuous single ECG monitor
8. Control systemic hypertension:
   Give propranolol 0.5 mg IV slowly, and further increments of 0.5 mg until a bradycardia results. In addition commence a Nitroprusside infusion @ 25μg/min (50 mg in 250 ml 5%

Dextrose), and titrate dose to maintain systolic blood pressure at 80–90 mmHg (as long as renal perfusion is maintained resulting in a urine output of >25 ml/h).

NB: Do not use Nitroprusside alone without additional beta blockade as this regimen will increase dp/dt_{max} and wall stress.

Or

Commence a Trimethephan infusion @ 1–2 mg/min (500 mg in 500 ml 5% Dextrose).

Or

Commence a Labetolol infusion @ 2 mg/min (200 mg in 200 ml 5% Dextrose).

9. Arrange for early investigation (aortography, CT, echocardiography as detailed above)

Chest pain in the patient with an aortic dissection is related to stretching of the vasa nervorum of the adventitia by the expanding haematoma. The restoration of normal blood pressure frequently alleviates the pain without additional analgesia. If necessary diamorphine 2.5–5.0 mg IV or morphine 5–10 mg IV may be needed.

DeBakey Type I/II (Stanford Type A) aortic dissections

1. *Acute*

   Operative intervention is the treatment of choice for this group of patients unless they are not surgical candidates on other grounds. Patients with a major neurological deficit (including paraplegia) or mesenteric infarction are probably best managed conservatively. Ideally, surgery is undertaken when the patient is haemodynamically stable and normotensive. The heart and great vessels are exposed by a median sternotomy and surgery is undertaken on low flow, low pressure total cardiopulmonary bypass with moderate hypothermia. A limited resection of the ascending aorta is undertaken to include the intimal tear, and a low-porosity Dacron tube graft is interposed using Teflon felt to reinforce the anastomoses. Depending in the site of the tear, coronary reimplantation may be necessary, but the aortic valve can be preserved in the majority (>80%) of cases. Operative mortality in experienced centres is 25–30%.

2. *Chronic*

   Chronic (>14 day) proximal dissections constitute <10% of the total and are associated with a favourable prognosis if managed conservatively. Strict blood pressure control is maintained after the acute event with an oral beta blocking agent (e.g. Propranolol, Atenolol) and a thiazide diuretic (e.g. bendrofluazide, hydrochlorothiazide). A combination alpha and beta blocking drug (e.g. Labetolol) is a satisfactory alternative, but oral vasodilators (e.g. hydrallazine, prazosin, captopril) should be avoided. Serial chest radiography, CT and echocardiography is undertaken to detect progression of the lesion. A more aggressive approach may become necessary.

DeBakey Type III (Stanford Type B) aortic dissections

1. *Acute*

There is controversy as to whether surgical or medical management is preferable in these patients. Most authorities favour conservative management (outlined above) with emphasis on strict blood pressure control. Even in the patient with a normal BP after the acute event beta blockade is advised in an attempt to reduce circumferential wall stress. Patients in this group are carefully followed with serial chest radiography, CT and echocardiography, and surgical intervention is advised on the following grounds:

a Extension of the dissecting haematoma on optimal medical therapy:
   (i) Increase in size on CXR, CT
   (ii) Clinical or echo evidence of aortic regurgitation
   (iii) Clinical signs of compromise of major branch artery (e.g. CVA, painful cold extremity, anuria etc.).
       NB: Surgical treatment is appropriate for all thoracic aneuryms >10 cm diameter as the incidence of subsequent rupture is high (75%).

b. Impending rupture of the dissection:
   (i) Acute saccular aneurysm on aortography
   (ii) Significant increase in size over a few hours (CXR, CT)
   (iii) Bleeding into the pericardiumn (echo), or pleural space (CXR, CT).

c. Inability to control BP and/or pain within 4 hours of onset (frequently related to renal ischaemia secondary to renal artery involvement in the dissection).

d. Marfan's syndrome.

Those that favour early surgery in this group point out that the hospital operative mortality is <15% in the patient without major complications, but this increases to 75% in the patient who has deteriorated as above.

2. *Chronic*

Appropriate management of these patients includes BP control and serial non-invasive investigations to evaluate progress of the dissection. Surgery is considered if there is development of a localised saccular aneurysm (2–14%), compression of a major branch artery by haematoma, or the aneurysm increases in diameter (>10 cm).

11. INFECTIVE ENDOCARDITIS

In the past, infective endocarditis was a disease of young adults, but currently the average age is 50–60 years with males affected more frequently than females (2:1). Approximately 300 new cases are notified annually in England and Wales. Factors responsible for the changing pattern of infective endocarditis include an increasing number of patients undergoing cardiac surgery, the reduction in the incidence of rheumatic fever, and an increase in intravenous drug abuse (particularly in the USA). Despite the availability of effective antibiotics the prognosis has not improved significantly in recent years with the overall case fatality rate remaining at 30%. Furthermore, the indiscriminate use of antibiotics has increased the frequency of culture negative endocarditis which is associated with an adverse prognosis.

Some types of endocarditis are more virulent than others, but as the natural history of endocarditis has been modified by antibiotics the terms 'acute' and 'chronic' are no longer applicable. Infective rather than bacterial endocarditis is the preferred term as a small but significant proportion of cases are non-bacterial. Non-infective endocarditis may be seen in the elderly and in patients with advanced malignancy (marantic endocarditis), and occasionally in association with systemic lupus erythematosus (Libman-Sachs endocarditis), or in other situations in which endothelial injury occurs without additional infection (e.g. indwelling central venous lines, cardiac catheterisation).

PATHOGENESIS

Micro-organisms gain entry to the blood stream by variety of routes, although the portal of entry can be determined in only one third of cases (Table 11.1). Less than 15% of patients give a history of dental treatment in the three months prior to clinical evidence of endocarditis.

Episodes of transient bacteraemia during dental treatment or other minor surgical procedures are a common occurrence, with no sequelae in most instances. However, areas of endothelial injury may provide a focus for the formation of a platelet-fibrin aggregate within which small numbers of circulating bacteria become entrapped and multiply.

Table 11.1 Infective endocarditis: portals of entry

	%
1. Dental treatment	<15
2. Genitourinary tract	4
3. Gastrointestinal	4
4. Respiratory	3
5. Skin	3
6. Cardiac surgery	3
7. Vascular surgery (non cardiac)	3
8. Drugs	1
9. Pregnancy	<1
10. Fractures	<1
11. Unknown	64

Endothelial damage results from turbulence (e.g. bicuspid aortic valve, pulmonary stenosis, mitral valve prolapse), and may be associated with high pressure interfaces (e.g. VSD, PDA, coarctation of the aorta, hypertrophic cardiomyopathy). 10–20% of adults with infective endocarditis have no known cardiac disease, whereas 50% of intravenous drug abusers have previously normal hearts.

Cardiac disease particularly susceptible to infective endocarditis:

1. Aortic valve disease (e.g. bicuspid aortic valve)
2. Mitral regurgitation
3. Prosthetic heart valves
4. Patent ductus arteriosus
5. Ventricular septal defect
6. Coarctation of the aorta
7. Marfan's syndrome.

An infected cardiac focus causes damage by three mechanisms:

1. *Tissue destruction*
   Multiplication of organisms results in tissue necrosis and abscess formation. Infection of the aortic valve causes severe regurgitation either by cusp rupture or perforation. Mitral regurgitation occurs secondary to cusp perforation or chordal rupture (especially to the anterior cusp). Other complications include abscess formation within the interventricular septum (which may involve the conduction system or progress to cause an acute VSD), rupture of a sinus of Valsalva aneurysm, and rarely direct pericardial invasion.
2. *Emboli*
   Septic emboli occur in 15–40% of patients and may involve any major vessel. Frequently emboli pass to the coronary, cerebral, renal or splenic vessels and the limbs may also be affected. Vegetations in fungal endocarditis are particularly large and friable. Patients with right sided disease can present with pulmonary emboli. Complications of septic emboli include mycotic aneurysm, abscess formation and infarction.

3. *Immune complex disease*
   Many of the classic clinical findings in infective endocarditis initially assumed to be due to microembolism are now thought to be related to endothelial damage caused by immune complex vasculitis. These include arthritis, tenosynovitis, Osler's nodes, Roth spots, Janeway lesions, subungal haemorrhages, glomerulonephritis, sterile meningitis and cerebritis. Typical findings include the presence of immune complexes in the serum, elevated immunoglobulins, positive rheumatoid factor, low levels of haemolytic complement and occasional false positive serology for syphilis.

The pathogenesis of some of the complications of infective endocarditis (e.g. clubbing, myocarditis) remains unclear.

MICRO-ORGANISMS

It is only with a knowledge of the organisms responsible for infective endocarditis that appropriate antibiotic treatment can be given (Tables 11.2 & 11.3). This is particularly important if therapy needs to be started early, prior to isolating the organism, due to haemodynamic deterioration; or alternatively, antibiotics have to be given empirically to the patient with culture negative endocarditis. The spectrum of infective endocarditis in IV drug abusers differs in that infection with Staphylococcus spp. occurs in 50%, Pseudomonas spp. in 15% and fungal (frequently Candida spp.) endocarditis in 5% of patients.

Table 11.2 Organisms causing infective endocarditis

	%	
1. Streptococcus spp.	60	(Streptococcus viridans 45%)
2. Staphylococcus spp.	20	
3. Bowel organisms	15	
4. Other bacteria	5	
5. Non-bacterial	<1	
6. Culture negative	10	

Table 11.3 Causes of culture negative endocarditis

1. Previous antibiotic treatment
2. Cell wall defective variants (e.g. L forms)
3. Anaerobic (e.g. bacteroides spp.), microaerophillic (e.g. some streptococcus spp.) and fastidious organisms (e.g. brucella spp.)
4. Non-bacterial (e.g. Coxiella burnetii or 'Q fever', Chlamydia psittaci, aspergillus spp., candida spp.)
5. 'Bacteria-free stage'. Rare. Occurs late in untreated infective endocarditis
6. Non-infective (thrombotic) endocarditis
7. Other diseases causing fever and emboli (e.g. LA myxoma)

SYMPTOMS

1. *Systemic illness*
   Due to the insidious nature and non-specific symptoms of infective endocarditis the diagnosis is frequently missed, and in retrospect many patients have been unwell for 4–8 weeks prior to the diagnosis being made. Typical symptoms are those of a 'viral illness' namely lassitude, general malaise, anorexia, weight loss, headache, sweats and rigors.
2. *Due to embolism*
   Any major artery may be affected by emboli. Involvement of the central nervous system may be apparent due to hemiparesis or visual disturbance. Abdominal symptoms result from a mesenteric embolism or splenic infarct (or abscess), and loin pain from renal infarction. Infected emboli from right-sided lesions cause pulmonary embolism, infarction and abscess formation.
3. *Due to immune complex deposition*
   Many of the peripheral manifestations of infective endocarditis result from immune complex deposition causing vascular injury; these include arthralgia, skin and eye lesions and symptoms of meningitis or cerebritis.
4. *Due to elevated pulmonary venous pressure*
   Breathlessness, orthopnoea and paroxysmal nocturnal dyspnoea may be sudden in onset due to acute mitral regurgitation (secondary to chordal rupture), severe aortic regurgitation or acute myocardial infarction due to a coronary embolism. Alternatively, symptoms can be progressive as a result of left ventricular decompensation caused by chronic aortic or mitral regurgitation or myocarditis.

CLINICAL SIGNS

Peripheral manifestations

1. *Asthenia*
   Evidence of weight loss, pallor (± uraemia).
2. *Fever*
   Typically low grade, but high fevers do occur particularly with staphylococcal disease.
   NB: Up to 15% of patients are afebrile throughout their illness (particularly the elderly).
3. *Anaemia*

4. *Petechiae (20–40%)*
Particularly frequently seen on the conjunctivae and the soft palate. Petechiae also occur in septicaemia (without endocarditis), SLE, and following cardio pulmonary bypass and are therefore non-specific. Petechiae with a pale centre are said to be a more reliable sign.

5. *Subungal ('splinter') haemorrhages (10%)*
Non-specific, occurring frequently in a hospital population, particularly the elderly. The proximal 'splinter' is a more reliable sign as the distal lesion is often related to trauma.

6. *Osler's nodes (10–20%)*
Small, painful, tender swellings most commonly in the finger pulp of the terminal phalanx. May be transient. Also occur rarely in SLE.

7. *Janeway lesions (rare)*
Small, non-tender red macular lesions that blanch on pressure. Usually occur on the palms or soles.

8. *Retinal haemorrhages (5–10%)*
Various non-specific types of haemorrhage occur in endocarditis including 'dot' and 'flame' haemorrhages. Roth spots are aggregates of cytoid bodies and are seen as an irregular halo with a white or yellow centre. Rarely, 'boat shaped' haemorrhages are visible.

9. *Clubbing (<15%)*
Seen less frequently than formerly. Aetiology unclear, but resolves with successful antibiotic treatment.

10. *Splenomegaly (30%)*
Mild to moderate splenomegaly. Tenderness suggests embolic splenic infarct or abscess.

11. *Haematuria and proteinuria*
Results from proliferative glomerulonephritis or renal infarction.

Cardiac manifestations

1. *Tachycardia*
Related to fever and anaemia. Atrial fibrillation is rare in infective endocarditis. Junctional or ventricular arrhythmias or intermittent atrioventricular block suggests a septal abscess.

2. *Murmurs*
New or changing murmurs are the classic feature of infective endocarditis. Involvement of the mitral (30–45%) and aortic valve (15–25%) is seen most frequently, and in the normal adult tricuspid disease is uncommon (<5%). In IV drug abusers the tricuspid valve is affected in 50% of patients. Pulmonary involvement is very rare. The characteristic signs

of mitral and aortic regurgitation may not be obvious due to the rapid onset of tissue destruction. It is not uncommon to see a patient with severe aortic or mitral regurgitation with no detectable murmurs. Peripheral features of aortic regurgitation (e.g. sharp upstroke, wide pulse pressure) are often inconspicuous. Other murmurs that may be detected include a 'flow' murmur across the left ventricular outflow tract related to fever and anaemia, the murmurs of a VSD or PDA in association with infective endocarditis, and the continuous murmur of a ruptured sinus of Valsalva aneurysm (usually in communication with the right atrium or right ventricle). Rarely, the bulky vegetations of fungal endocarditis may obstruct the orifice of the aortic, mitral or tricuspid valves.

3. *Acute pulmonary oedema*
   Pulmonary oedema in association with infective endocarditis is poorly tolerated. The rapidity of onset of aortic regurgitation in the relatively non-compliant left ventricle of normal volume results in early pulmonary oedema. Similarly, sudden mitral regurgitation secondary to chordal rupture in association with a normal sized left atrium causes a sudden elevation in left atrial pressure and early decompensation. The mortality of the patient in pulmonary oedema may approach 90%, similarly the results of valve replacement in this group are poor.

4. *Pericarditis*
   Mostly occurs as an immunological complication of infective endocarditis, rarely as a result of direct invasion (e.g. ruptured sinus of Valsalva aneurysm), or secondary to uraemia.

5. *Myocardial abscess*
   Intracardiac abscesses may involve the interventricular septum as a result of extension of infection from the aortic valve, aortic annulus or atrioventricular valve ring. Staphylococcal infection is the most common cause. Complications include progressive atrioventricular block and ventricular septal defect. Abscesses may also develop following an infected coronary embolism, or cause sudden death from cardiac rupture and tamponade.

Neurological manifestations

In 10–15% of patients with infective endocarditis the presenting symptom is neurological, and CNS complications are present in 15–30% of all patients during the course of their illness. Mortality in this group is double that of those without neurological involvement.

Neurological complications include:
1. Cerebral infarction (embolism or haemorrhage)
2. Mycotic aneurysm
3. Cerebral abscess
4. Seizures
5. Meningitis
   CSF shows elevated protein, increased polymorphs, but
   normal glucose and sterile. Rarely bacterial meningitis
   develops as a complication of pneumococcal or staphylococcal
   infection.
6. Cerebritis
7. Subarachnoid haemorrhage
8. Mononeuritis

INVESTIGATIONS

1. *Haematology*
   A high ESR (50–100 mm/1h) is typical. A mild leucocytosis
   is frequently seen with a left shift (immature forms), and
   histiocytes in the peripheral blood. A normochromic
   normocytic anaemia is usually present. Rarely a haemolytic
   anaemia occurs, and thrombocytopaenia can result from
   disseminated intravascular coagulation. Examination of the
   'buffy' coat from peripheral blood may reveal the causative
   organism.
2. *Blood culture*
   Bacteraemia in infective endocarditis is continuous,
   therefore blood cultures timed to coincide with peaks of
   fever are unnecessary. Nor is there any advantage in taking
   samples of arterial blood, central venous blood or bone
   marrow for culture. The skin is carefully cleaned and 2–6
   sets of blood cultures drawn over a 30–60 minute period
   will suffice. Aerobic and anaerobic cultures are set up, and
   additional cultures containing penicillinase if penicillin has
   been administered within the previous 48 hours. It is
   important to add enough blood (10 ml) to the correct
   quantity of culture medium (100 ml). A close liaison
   between the clinician and microbiologist will ensure
   optimum conditions of incubation, and will also be beneficial
   in the monitoring of antibiotic therapy. In cases of culture
   positive bacterial endocarditis the organism will be isolated
   from the first blood culture in 60–90% of cases. Adequate
   growth usually takes <48 hours.

3. *Serology*
Blood is drawn for Coxiella and Chlamydia complement fixation tests.

4. *Immunological studies*
Circulating immune complexes are present in the serum of 80–95% of patients with infective endocarditis, and levels of haemolytic complement (C_3, C_4, CH_{50}) are reduced in 30% of patients. Immunoglobulins are elevated, and 50% of patients have a positive rheumatoid factor. False positive serology for syphilis (VDRL) may occur.

5. *Urinalysis*
Microscopic haematuria is a useful indicator of active endocarditis. Red cell casts and proteinuria indicate focal or proliferative glomerulonephritis. Macroscopic haematuria is seen in renal infarction.
NB: Microscopic haematuria in a patient on anticoagulants with a prosthetic valve is *not* a normal finding. Investigation for haemolysis and endocarditis is warranted.

6. *Chest radiograph*
Abnormalities of the chest radiograph are non-specific. Features of pulmonary oedema are an ominous sign, and the relative normality of cardiac size in association with acute pulmonary oedema may be striking. Aortic valve calcification is best seen on the lateral projection, and confirmed by fluoroscopy. Fluoroscopy is also useful in the investigation of abnormal prosthetic valve movement but the specificity of this technique is low. Pulmonary abscesses or infarction are complications of right-sided disease and tomography or chest CT can confirm the plain CXR findings.

7. *Electrocardiogram*
Sinus tachycardia accompanies the systemic illness. Atrial fibrillation is rare. Abnormalities of conduction or changes in electrical axis indicate formation of a septal abscess. Serial ECG's should be recorded and compared in order to identify this complication. Rarely, a coronary embolism will result in acute myocardial infarction with typical ECG features.

8. *Nuclear imaging*
Although [67]Gallium scanning has been used in the investigation of active cardiac infection it cannot be recommended as a useful diagnostic procedure at present. Liver and spleen scanning may reveal evidence of embolic infarction or abscess formation.

9. *M-mode and cross-sectional echocardiography*
All patients suspected of having infective endocarditis should

undergo serial examination by echocardiography. Not only can ultrasound frequently identify vegetations with certainty and provide information on the haemodynamic consequences of valvular dysfunction, but information gained from echocardiography may make the optimal timing of surgical intervention easier.

Due to difficulties visualising vegetations of <3 mm diameter, the sensitivity of echocardiography in detecting vegetations is approximately 50–60%. Associated mitral or tricuspid prolapse secondary to chordal rupture may be apparent, and prolapse of an aortic cusp may also be seen. Visualisation of abscesses involving the interventricular septum and aortic root are best appreciated by the cross-sectional technique. Changes in left ventricular dimensions and filling rate are determined by M-mode echocardiography, and the presence of premature mitral closure (i.e. closure of the mitral valve prior to the QRS complex, indicative of an elevated LVEDP) is an indication for urgent surgery.

Echocardiography cannot provide information on the sterility of vegetations, nor on the adequacy of treatment. Little information is available on the natural history of vegetations visualised by echocardiography (vis à vis embolisation), and the appearance of large vegetations in the patient who is asymptomatic having successfully completed a course of antibiotics may be alarming. In prosthetic endocarditis the high echodensity of the prosthesis itself makes recognition of adjacent vegetations difficult or impossible.

10. *Cardiac catheterisation*
    Patients undergoing antibiotic treatment can be monitored by clinical examination and echocardiography. Cardiac catheterisation may be required prior to operative intervention in order to document an intracardiac shunt, or demonstrate coronary artery anatomy. The risk of dislodging a vegetation must be considered.

TREATMENT OF INFECTIVE ENDOCARDITIS

The successful treatment of the patient with infective endocarditis remains a therapeutic challenge. The choice of antibiotic, the correct dose, the route of administration, the length of treatment and the appropriate use and timing of surgery are all important determinants of a favourable result.

Antibiotics

Although classical teaching advocates 6 weeks of intravenous antibiotics for all patients with infective endocarditis, it is preferable to administer the appropriate regimen for each organism (Table 11.4). Uncomplicated streptococcal endocarditis may only require 2 weeks treatment, whereas staphylococcal infection may require antibiotics for 6–8 weeks. In general, bactericidal rather than bacteriostatic antibiotics are favoured except in special circumstances (e.g. Coxiella). An indwelling central venous line (renewed with an aseptic technique each week) is preferred, although some authorities favour rotating peripheral sites. Antibiotics should be administered by bolus, rather than by continuous infusion. Oral antibiotic regimens can only be recommended in certain circumstances, usually after an initial two week course of intravenous therapy.

Adequacy of antibiotic dosage is monitored by means of the serum bactericidal titre (SBT), in which the organism is exposed to the patient's own serum (containing the antibiotic) at increasing dilutions. An SBT of 1:8 or greater is acceptable, and the dose of antibiotic can be altered accordingly. Even when an optimal antibiotic regimen has been continued for six weeks, cultures taken from valve tissue will grow the organism in >30% of cases.

If a patient is transferred to a specialist cardiac unit for further

Table 11.4 Specific antibiotic regimens

Strep viridans	Benzyl Penicillin 3–4 mega units IV every 6 h + Gentamicin 1.5 mg/kg IV every 8 h
Staph spp.	Flucloxacillin 1–2 g IV every 4 h + Gentamicin 1.5 mg/kg IV every 8 h + Fucidic acid 500 mg IV every 8 h
Strep faecalis	Ampicillin 2 g IV every 4 h + Gentamicin 1.5 mg/kg IV every 8 h
Pseudomonas spp.	Azlocillin 5 g IV every 8 h + Gentamicin 1.5 mg/kg IV every 8 h
Candida spp.	Amphotericin 0.25–1.5 mg/day IV (max total dose 1.5–3.0 g) + 5-fluorocytosine 50–150 mg/kg PO every 6 h
Coxiella burnetti ('Q fever')	Tetracycline 1 g IV every 12 h or Cotrimoxazole 10 ml IV every 12 h (Trimethoprim 160 mg + Sulphamethoxazole 800 mg)
Culture negative	Ampicillin 2 g IV every 4 h Flucloxacillin 1–2 g IV every 4 h Gentamicin 1.5 mg/kg IV every 8 h

management it is useful to send a specimen of the organism so that the SBT can continue to be monitored following transfer. For patients allergic to the penicillins, Vancomycin 15 mg/kg every 12 hours can be substituted. Alternatively, the patient can be desensitised. Side effects of high dose penicillins include seizures and thrombocytopaenia. Aminoglycosides are monitored with peak and trough levels (Gentamicin/Tobramycin trough <2 mg/l, peak 5–12 mg/l), and total dose may be an important factor in causing vestibular damage. If renal function is impaired the interval between doses is increased. These drugs should be used with great care in the elderly. Fucidic acid is contraindicated in the patient with hepatic dysfunction, and amphotericin is nephrotoxic. Occasionally a low grade fever will develop during antibiotic treatment which may either represent a failure to control the infective process or a drug reaction.

Surgery

During the course of the illness 10–20% of patients will require cardiac surgery (Table 11.5). The correct timing of surgical intervention in these patients is critical. Not only is the operative mortality reduced when elective rather than emergency valve replacement is undertaken (<10% vs>30%), but the incidence of reoperation is considerably less in the patients undergoing elective surgery.There is no evidence to suggest that early operation (prior to completing a course of antibiotics) results in an increased incidence of recurrent infection. The patient with aortic regurgitation is at particular risk from developing low cardiac output, pulmonary oedema and multiple organ failure. Similarly, the severity of mitral regurgitation complicating chordal rupture only improves at the expense of left ventricular dilatation. In general the patient with 'aggressive' endocarditis (e.g. staphylococcal, gram negative) is more likely to require surgery than the patient with streptococcal infection. Biological valves are favoured in patients with infective endocarditis.

Antibiotic prophylaxis
Data supporting the routine use of prophylactic antibiotics is anecdotal and inconclusive. Transient bacteraemia frequently complicates minor surgical procedures although only a small proportion of susceptible

Table 11.5 Indications for surgical intervention

1. Moderate/severe aortic or mitral regurgitation
2. Multiple pulmonary or systemic emboli
3. Septal abscess
4. Sinus of Valsalva aneurysm
5. Prosthetic endocarditis
6. Fungal endocarditis
7. Other non-bacterial infective endocarditis (e.g. Coxiella)
8. Relapse or recurrence of endocarditis (<6/12)
9. Correction of congenital heart disease following infective endocarditis (e.g. PDA, VSD, coarctation of the aorta)
10. No response to antibiotics

patients develop infective endocarditis. Furthermore, the administration of the appropriate antibiotics at the correct time, by the correct route in the correct dose is difficult to achieve in outpatient practice.

Antibiotic prophylaxis is advisable for the following groups of patients:

1. Congenital heart disease (including bicuspid aortic valve)
2. Congenital heart disease 'corrected' with foreign material (e.g. patch, conduit)
3. Rheumatic heart disease
4. Mitral annulus calcification
5. Mitral valve prolapse
6. Hypertrophic cardiomyopathy
7. Valvular prostheses.

Prophylactic antibiotic regimens

1. *Dental treatment*
   Extractions, scaling and root canal work under local anaesthesia:
   Amoxycillin 3 g PO 1 hour prior to surgery
   (<10 years 1.5 g, <5 years 0.75 g)
   or: Erythromycin stearate 1.5 g PO 1–2 hours prior to surgery then 0.5 g 6 hours later (if allergic to penicillin).

2. *Dental treatment*
   In the patient who has had penicillin within the last month, or who has a prosthetic valve, or who has had previous endocarditis, or who requires treatment under general anaesthesia.

3. *Genitourinary*
   Cystoscopy, urethral dilatation, prostatectomy, catheterisation with infected urine, transrectal biopsy prostate.

4. *Obstetrics and gynaecology*
   Vaginal delivery, insertion/removal IUCD, D&C, only with prosthetic valves.

5. *Gastroenterology*
   Panendoscopy, proctoscopy, sigmoidoscopy, colonoscopy, barium enema, only with prosthetic valves.

6. *Upper respiratory tract*
   Tonsillectomy.

Patients in Groups 2–6 should receive:
   Amoxycillin 1 g + Gentamicin 120 mg IM prior to induction then Amoxycillin 0.5 g IM/PO 6 hours later
   (<10 years Amoxycillin 0.5 + 0.25 g, Gentamicin 2 mg/kg)
   or: Vancomycin 1 g slow IV infusion 20–30 min prior to induction +Gentamicin 120 mg IM
   (<10 years Vancomycin 20 mg/kg)

12. MYOCARDITIS

Due to the difficulty in making an accurate clinical diagnosis of myocarditis, much controversy exists concerning the incidence, treatment and prognosis of the condition. It has become clear that there is overlap between idiopathic dilated cardiomyopathy and myocarditis and that the two conditions can only be diagnosed with certainty by means of endomyocardial biopsy. Endomyocardial biopsy confirms the clinical impression of myocarditis in only 20–30% of cases; conversely in one series of patients with biopsy proven myocarditis the diagnosis had only been considered in 10% of cases. Even the histological diagnosis of myocarditis is complicated by the lack of concensus among pathologists as to what degree of inflammatory infiltrate constitutes a myocarditis. These difficulties account for the apparent lack of agreement as to the appropriate management of these patients.

AETIOLOGY

Inflammation of the myocardium may complicate a number of infections and infestations, or result from physical injury due to radiation or cardiotoxic drugs (Table 12.1). Furthermore, myocarditis is a frequently unrecognised complication of systemic infections supported by histological evidence of myocarditis in 5–10% of routine postmortem examinations. Myocarditis is found in up to 5% of young patients dying suddenly (see Ch. 16).

Table 12.1 Causes of myocarditis

1. Viruses (e.g. Coxsackie A & B, Echo, Infuenza, Hepatitis A, EBV, CMV)
2. Mycoplasma pneumoniae
3. Chlamydia psittaci
4. Rickettsia (e.g. Typhus)
5. Bacteria (e.g. Diphtheria)
6. Spirochaetes (e.g. Leptospirosis)
7. Fungi (e.g. Aspergillus)
8. Protozoa (e.g. Trypanosoma cruzi, Toxoplasma gondii)
9. Drugs (e.g. phenothiazines, lithium, catecholamines, cyclophosphamide, daunorubicin, adriamycin)
10. Acute rejection following cardiac transplantation

193

SYMPTOMS

Most patients with viral myocarditis are asymptomatic and suffer no myocardial dysfunction either at the time of the acute infection or subsequently. What is not clear is why occasional patients sustain myocardial damage following viral infection or why others appear to develop a dilated cardiomyopathy later. Biopsy evidence of viral infection (e.g. viral inclusions) are rarely seen; the lag period of several weeks between the acute infection and the abnormality of cardiac function lends support to the concept of an immune basis to the condition. In the few patients who develop a florid myocarditis symptoms are related to impaired systolic function and a raised pulmonary venous pressure (see Ch. 5) as well as abnormal diastolic function resulting in a reduction in myocardial compliance. Chest pain may occur with pericardial involvement.

PHYSICAL SIGNS

1. General malaise, myalgia and fever (usually resolved)
2. Elevated venous pressure
3. Sinus tachycardia
4. Third heart sound or gallop rhythm
5. Pulmonary oedema

INVESTIGATIONS

1. *Blood tests*
   Elevated white cell count (typically lymphocytosis). Paired sera may indicate recent viral infection by complement fixation or haemagglutination inhibition. Virus may be isolated from throat washings, blood or faeces, but rarely from myocardium. As creatine kinase (CPK) may be released from the myocardium or skeletal muscle, monitoring CPK.MB is more specific as an indicator of myocardial damage.
2. *Electrocardiography*
   Abnormalities of the ECG may be the only manifestation of myocarditis in a patient with a viral illness. Early in the course of the illness the ECG manifestations of pericarditis (see Ch. 13) may predominate. T wave inversion may be dramatic and depending on the distribution of the changes, differentiation from acute myocardial infarction may be difficult.

Transient AV block and ventricular arrhythmias are a significant cause of morbidity and mortality. Holter monitoring should be undertaken in all patients with symptomatic myocarditis.

3. *Chest radiograph*
   Initially the cardiothoracic ratio may be normal with evidence of an elevated pulmonary venous pressure and interstitial oedema. Later all cardiac chambers become dilated.

4. *M-mode and cross-sectional echocardiography*
   Early in the disease, myocardial oedema may cause apparent hypertrophy with an appearance similar to a restrictive cardiomyopathy (see p. 127). In severe cases ventricular dilatation is associated with global impairment of systolic function indistinguishable from idiopathic dilated cardiomyopathy (see p. 119). Thrombi may be visible in either ventricle.

5. *Cardiac catheterisation*
   Invasive assessment may be required to exclude coronary artery disease and is a necessary prerequisite for endomyocardial biopsy.

6. *Endomyocardial biopsy*
   Cardiac biopsy is important in the assessment of the patient with possible myocarditis and is mandatory prior to commencing immunosuppressive drugs. Morbidity from cardiac biopsy is low in experienced hands there but are a number of problems associated with the technique, not least of which is the interpretatioin of the histological appearances of the specimens. Myocarditis is focal and in order to avoid sampling error at least five specimens should be taken from the left or right ventricle. Criteria for the histological diagnosis of myocarditis are listed in Table 12.2.

7. *[67]Gallium scanning*
   [67]Gallium citrate has a high affinity for activated T cells and preliminary data suggest that myocardial uptake of this radionuclide may be a useful addition to endomyocardial

---

Table 12.2 Criteria for the histological diagnosis of myocarditis

1. *Leucocytic infiltrate*
   Predominately lymphocytes and monocytes. At least 5 cells should be identified per high power field as occasional lymphocytes are seen in normal myocardium.

2. *Myocyte necrosis*
   Destruction of myocytes must accompany the inflammatory infiltrate. Myocyte necrosis may be focal or diffuse.

3. *Fibrosis*
   Myocarditis may resolve or organise. Fibrosis alone is non-specific and does not constitute a myocarditis.

biopsy in the diagnosis and monitoring of patients with myocarditis.

MANAGEMENT

1. *No treatment*
   Most patients requiree no specific treatment other than monitoring the ECG for arrhythmias or conduction disturbance, and serial echocardiograms are used to follow ventricular function.`

2. *Immunosuppression*
   If endomyocardial biopsy reveals a severe myocarditis or there is evidence of haemodynamic compromise, immunosuppression is commenced as prednisolone 1.25 mg/kg/day tapering over a 6 month period depending on clinical and histological response, together with azathioprine 2 mg/kg/day.

3. *Inotropic support*
   Evidence of cardiogenic shock is treated in the usual way (see p. 38).

4. *Cardiac transplantation*
   In a small subgroup of patients, early cardiac transplantation offers the only chance of survival.

13. PERICARDIAL DISEASE

ANATOMY

The heart is enclosed in the pericardial cavity which comprises a fibrous sac (parietal pericardium), and a thin layer of loose connective tissue on the epicardial surface of the heart (visceral pericardium). The parietal pericardium is fused to the adventitia of the great vessels. A reflection of parietal pericardium, the oblique sinus, lies behind the left atrium, and the transverse sinus lies posterior to the great vessels and anterior to the atria.

Varying amounts of fat underly the visceral pericardium (i.e. between the visceral pericardium and the myocardium). Within the pericardial sac, 30–50 ml fluid act as 'lubrication'. Pathological consequences of fluid accumulation within the pericardial space relate to the rate of accumulation rather than the absolute amount of fluid.

PATHOLOGY

Inflammation of the pericardium is characterised by a cellular reaction and an exudate of fibrin and fluid. In viral disease the pericardial reaction is mild. In bacterial pericarditis an intense polymorphonuclear leucocyte response is seen, and in tuberculous pericarditis there is a mononuclear infiltrate with later development of dense fibrosis and constriction.

ACUTE PERICARDITIS

Aetiology

Acute pericarditis may occur in isolation or as part of a systemic illness. Pericarditis may also be seen at autopsy as an incidental finding. Many causes of pericarditis have been identified (Table 13.1), but in clinical practice viral or idiopathic pericarditis account for most cases out of

Table 13.1 Causes of acute pericarditis

1. Infection (bacterial, viral, tuberculous, parasitic)
2. Neoplasia (metastatic, contiguous spread, primary pericardial)
3. Metabolic disorders (uraemia, hypothyroidism, hyperuricaemia)
4. Connective tissue disease (rheumatoid, rheumatic fever, SLE, PAN)
5. Cardiovascular disease (acute myocardial infarction including Dressler's, aortic dissection)
6. Trauma (cardiothoracic surgery, chest injuries, DXT)
7. Drug induced (hydrallazine, penicillin, isoniazid)

hospital. Serological evidence of a viral infection may be lacking, and many of these cases are labelled 'idiopathic'. Important causes of pericarditis in hospitalised patients include uraemia, neoplasia, post myocardial infarction, and post cardiotomy pericarditis. Bacterial pericarditis is seen as a complication of septicaemia, infective endocarditis, thoracic surgery or trauma.

Clinical history

1. *Prodromal illness*
   Symptoms of a flu-like illness may precede the onset of viral pericarditis.
2. *Pain*
   Severe chest pain is characteristic of acute pericarditis. Low retrosternal pain radiating to the neck, shoulders or dorsal spine, aggravated by movement, and relieved by leaning forward is typical. In viral and connective tissue disease, pleuritic pain may also be present. Only 25% of patients with purulent pericarditis experience chest pain.
3. *Breathlessness*
   Results from an inability to take a deep breath (because of pain) or an increased left atrial pressure in cardiac tamponade.
4. *Constitutional disturbance*
   Anorexia, general malaise, night sweats, and a cough may dominate the clinical picture particularly in purulent or tuberculous pericarditis in which pericardial involvement complicates systemic infection.
5. *Underlying condition*
   Depending on the cause of the pericarditis, features of the underlying condition may be apparent (e.g. weight loss in neoplasia and tuberculosis, rash or arthralgia in connective tissue disease etc.).

Physical signs

1. *Related to viral or bacterial illness*
   e.g. fever.

2. *Venous pressure*

   In uncomplicated acute pericarditis the venous pressure is normal; an elevated venous pressure indicates an accumulation of pericardial fluid and incipient tamponade.

3. *Pericardial friction rub*

   Friction rubs may be difficult to hear because they are transient, well localised, and change in character with position. They are best heard at the lower left sternal border on full inspiration. A two component to and fro rub is heard in most patients, coinciding with atrial and ventricular systole. In up to 50% of patients an additional component can be detected in early diastole at the time of rapid ventricular filling. Mild exercise may make detection of a pericardial rub easier. It should be noted that a pericardial rub can still be heard in some patients with large pericardial effusions.

Investigations

1. *Blood tests*

   Routine blood tests should include a full blood count differential, ESR, viral screen (I + II), mycoplasma titre and blood cultures. In viral pericarditis a lymphocytosis is typical, whereas in a bacterial infection polymorphonuclear leucocytes predominate. Leucopaenia may be indicative of malignancy, tuberculosis or systemic lupus erythematosus. An elevated ESR is non-specific finding. In uraemic pericarditis the blood urea is usually very high. CPK.MB may be elevated in all forms of pericarditis and is *not* a reliable method of differentiating pericarditis from myocardial infarction.

   Viruses causing pericarditis include Coxsackie B4 and B6, echovirus, influenza, EB virus, adenovirus, varicella and hepatitis B. The spectrum of organisms causing purulent pericarditis has changed in recent years. Currently, gram negative bacilli account for 30% of infections, streptococcus pneumoniae 20%, and staphylococcal spp. 10%; 85% of infections are caused by a single organism. In paediatric patients, staphylococcal spp and haemophilus influenzae are the two most common organisms.

2. *Electrocardiogram*

   Sinus tachycardia is a frequent non-specific finding. Transient 'supraventricular' arrhythmias are uncommon, occurring in <25% of patients.

   In contrast to acute myocardial infarction the ECG manifestations of acute pericarditis are generalised (with no reciprocal changes) and are limited to the ST-T segment.

Abnormalities of the QRS complex are indicative of myocardial disease (e.g. acute myocardial infarction). Widespread ST segment elevation (concave upwards) is seen throughout the limb and precordial leads (except aVr and Vl). Initially the T waves are upright, but after a few days when the ST segments return to the isoelectric line the T waves flatten and become inverted. Unlike the repolarisation changes in acute myocardial infarction on the T waves invert *after* the ST segments normalise. Recording serial ECGs may be useful as the initial ST segment elevation may be missed. Less than 10% of patients with acute pericarditis have a normal ECG throughout their illness.

3. *Chest radiograph*
   This may be normal in uncomplicated pericarditis. Globular enlargement of the cardiac silhouette occurs when there is a significant pericardial effusion, but as this finding is non-specific the diagnosis is best confirmed by echocardiography. Areas of linear atelectasis and small pleural effusions are not uncommon.

4. *M-mode and cross-sectional echocardiography*
   Cross-sectional echocardiography is a rapid, accurate and simple method of confirming and quantitating a pericardial effusion, and differentiates enlargement of the cardiac silhouette due to LV dilatation from pericardial effusion. The presence of an echo-free space behind the LV cavity (but not behind the left atrium due to the oblique sinus) on M-mode echocardiography is diagnostic of a pericardial effusion but does not allow accurate localisation nor quantitation of the fluid. In uncomplicated pericarditis a small effusion may be seen (<100 ml) in the posterior pericardial space behind the LV. Slight pericardial thickening or adhesions may also be apparent and the irregular appearance of neoplasia is very characteristic.

Differential diagnosis

1. *Acute myocardial infarction*
   Possible prior history of angina. Rub absent early in myocardial infarction. QRS abnormalities and specific pattern of ST elevation with reciprocal changes. Cardiac enzymes unreliable, but enzyme release is greater after infarction.

2. *Aortic dissection*
   Pericardial effusion may complicate aortic dissection. Severe chest pain radiating through to the back. Shock. Absent or delayed pulses. Aortic regurgitation. Wide mediastinum on chest radiography, confirm with echocardiography, thoracic CT or aortography.

3. *Respiratory infection*
   Systemic features of pericarditis (e.g. fever, cough and sputum) may be mistaken for a respiratory infection. This mistake is compounded by hearing a friction rub (thought to be pleural in origin), and finding an abnormal chest radiograph (linear atelectasis and pleural effusions). An ECG will usually confirm pericarditis.

4. *Pulmonary embolism*
   In the post-cardiac surgical patient differentiating pulmonary embolism from acute pericarditis may be difficult. Again, the ECG is helpful in cases of pericarditis, and a ventilation-perfusion lung scan may indicate pulmonary embolism, although interpretation is difficult in the post-surgical patient. Pulmonary arteriography may be necessary. Inappropriate anticoagulation of a patient with pericarditis may cause catastrophic cardiac tamponade.

5. *Pneumothorax or pneumomediastinum*
   A spontaneous pneumothorax causing air to track medially around the hilum of the lung (pneumomediastinum) can cause referred pain similar in distribution to the pain of pericarditis. Clinical evidence of surgical emphysema may be apparent and the chest radiograph usually confirms the diagnosis.

Management

1. *Aspirin*
   As soon as the diagnosis is suspected Aspirin 600–1200 mg every four hours is given by mouth. Symptomatic relief may be satisfactory, but frequently additional medication is required.

2. *Non-steroidal anti-inflammatory agents (NSAID)*
   Indomethacin 50–200 mg daily, Naproxen 250–500 mg twice daily, or one of the other NSAID may be effective in some patients particularly those who cannot tolerate aspirin.

3. *Corticosteroids*
   If pain and fever have not subsided within 24–48 hours, the patient should be started on prednisolone 20 mg four times daily. High doses of steroids are rapidly effective in the majority of cases. After 7–10 days of treatment the steroids are gradually withdrawn by means of a tapering schedule. Steroid withdrawal may be facilitated by continuing treatment with other anti-inflammatory agents. Pericardiectomy should be considered in the few patients in whom steroid withdrawal is not possible.

4. *Antibiotics*
   In bacterial pericarditis the infecting organism may be

isolated from the blood or pericardial aspirate. High dose broad spectrum bacteriacidal antibiotics are commenced prior to isolating the organism. A gram stain on a sample of pericardial fluid may be diagnostic. Direct pericardial instillation of antibiotics is not required as therapeutic concentrations of antibiotics reach the inflamed pericardium. Surgical drainage is frequently necessary in these very sick patients.

Prognosis

A favourable outcome is seen in most cases of viral or idiopathic pericarditis within 2–6 weeks. Relapse may occur if steroid withdrawal is too rapid, and these patients require a very slow steroid taper over 3–6 months. Recurrent acute pericarditis is seen in <5% of patients but may be difficult to manage. Treatment should be recommenced as for the initial episode, but a proportion of this subgroup will require pericardiectomy which is effective in 80–90% of cases. An episode of acute pericarditis precedes the development of constrictive or effusive-constrictive pericarditis in the minority of patients (see p. 205).

PERICARDIAL TAMPONADE

Prompt recognition of pericardial tamponade can be life saving. A high index of suspicion together with appropriate non-invasive investigation (i.e. echocardiography) allows a rapid diagnosis to be made in the majority of patients.

Aetiology

Any cause of acute pericarditis can result in an accumulation of fluid sufficient to cause pericardial tamponade. Common causes of tamponade in hospitalised patients include malignancy, uraemia, post cardiac surgery and as a complication of cardiac catheterisation. Use of anticoagulants (e.g. in acute myocardial infarction) may provoke haemorrhagic effusions in some patients.

Pathophysiology

Cardiac tamponade is caused by a limitation in ventricular diastolic filling due to an increase in intrapericardial pressure as a consequence of pericardial fluid accumulation. Ultimately when intrapericardial pressure equals right atrial pressure circulation ceases. In acute tamponade the pericardial cavity can accomodate less than 500 ml of fluid before haemodynamic embarrassment is evident. In chronic disease, considerable pericardial dilatation occurs such that an effusion may reach 2–3 litres in volume.

Factors affecting the development of pericardial tamponade include:

1. Time period over which fluid accumulates
2. Degree of associated pericardial thickening (which reduces pericardial distensibility)
3. Presence of left ventricular hypertrophy
4. Circulating blood volume.

Clinical history

Clinical features of pericardial tamponade are those of 'shock' or circulatory collapse. In acute tamponade, the history relates to a sudden reduction in cardiac output which causes restlessness, confusion and breathlessness terminating in cardiac arrest within a few minutes. Symptoms of chronic tamponade are insidious; lethargy, weight loss, anorexia and breathlessness are the dominant features. Chest pain with the features of pericarditis occur in some patients (e.g. with malignancy or tuberculosis).

Physical signs

1. *'Shock'*
   Systemic hypotension, tachycardia and tachypnoea are evident. Because of the short history pallor and cool extremities may not be present.
2. *Elevated venous pressure*
   Marked elevation of the jugular venous pressure. Damped waveform with a prominent 'x' descent and absent 'y' descent.
3. *Pulsus paradoxus*
   Exaggeration of the normal change in systemic arterial pressure with respiration. During inspiration the pulse pressure falls due to a decrease in systolic pressure with little change in diastolic pressure. In normal subjects this reduction in pulse pressure is less than 10 mmHg, and 15 mmHg or more of arterial paradox is pathological. Arterial paradox is not specific for cardiac tamponade as it has been demonstrated in patients with pericardial constriction, restrictive cardiomyopathy, pulmonary embolism, severe airflow obstruction (e.g. bronchial asthma), hypovolaemic shock and in patients with tense ascites. Pathophysiology of arterial paradox is complex but two mechanisms are important:
   a. Changes in intrathoracic pressure affect systemic venous return

   b. Left and right ventricles compete for the available space
   within the pericardial cavity.

Investigations

   1. *Electrocardiography*
   Pendular swinging of the heart within the pericardial effusion
   causes phasic alteration in the amplitude of the R wave
   (electrical alternans). Other ECG features of pericarditis or
   pericardial constriction may be present.
   2. *Chest radiograph*
   Chronic pericardial effusions cause an increase in the
   cardiothoracic ratio and the cardiac silhouette takes on a
   globular appearance. In acute pericardial effusion the
   appearance of the heart may be unremarkable and a normal
   chest radiograph does not exclude a diagnosis of cardiac
   tamponade.
   3. *Echocardiography*
   Cross-sectional echocardiography can rapidly confirm the
   presence of a large pericardial effusion, but the diagnosis of
   cardiac tamponade by echocardiography is more difficult. In
   practice this is of little consequence as a patient who has
   collapsed and is shown to have a large pericardial effusion
   warrants immediate pericardial aspiration. The heart is seen
   to swing to and fro within the pericardial fluid (in time with
   the electrical alternans). Features of tamponade include
   diastolic collapse of the right ventricle, early systolic notching
   of the anterior right ventricular wall and sudden posterior
   movement of the interventricular septum on inspiration.
   4. *Cardiac catheterisation*
   This is not indicated in the management of acute cardiac
   tamponade.

Management

   1. *Pericardial aspiration*
   Details of this procedure can be found in Chapter 20.
   2. *Surgical intervention*
   Pericardectomy or formation of a pericardial window may be
   required in patients with recurrent pericardial effusions; this
   allows the pericardial fluid to drain into the thoracic cavity
   where it is absorbed via the pleura and lymphatics.

CONSTRICTIVE PERICARDITIS

The correct identification of pericardial constriction, and the differentiation between the patient suffering from constrictive pericarditis or restrictive cardiomyopathy is important because surgical intervention may be curative in pericardial constriction.

Aetiology

Some of the more common causes of pericardial constriction are listed in Table 13.2. Any cause of acute pericarditis may subsequently result in constrictive pericarditis. In the West, mediastinal irradiation has become one of the most frequent causes of pericardial constriction. Irradiation is used for the treatment of lymphoma and most patients developing constriction have received in excess of 4000 rads to the mediastinum. Constriction may follow months or years after irradiation. Other sequelae of radiation include coronary artery disease and pulmonary fibrosis. In the Third World, tuberculosis still accounts for at least 50% of patients (although the organism is seldom isolated), whereas in the UK the cause of constriction is unknown in the majority of cases. Rarely, constrictive pericarditis may be congenital.

Pathophysiology

Pericardial constriction is usually a diffuse process which limits volume expansion of the ventricles, particularly in late diastole. Occasionally, discrete plaques or bands of fibrosis or calcification may mimic valvular heart disease, by impeding inflow or outflow to one or other ventricle.

Clinical history

1. *General malaise*
   Chronic disability, fatigue, anorexia and weight loss characterise the insidious onset of pericardial constriction. Low cardiac output, hepatic and gut congestion account for most of these non-specific symptoms.

Table 13.2 Causes of constrictive pericarditis

1. Idiopathic
2. Tuberculosis
3. Bacterial or fungal infection
4. Uraemia
5. Connective tissue disease (rheumatoid, SLE)
6. Neoplasia
7. Deep X-ray therapy
8. Following haemopericardium (cardiac surgery, trauma etc.)
9. Following acute pericarditis (see Table 13.1)

2. *Breathlessness*
A fixed cardiac output causes exertional breathlessness;
splinting of the diaphragms by ascites and pleural effusions
may also contribute to the shortness of breath. Orthopnoea
and nocturnal dyspnoea are not features of pericardial
constriction.

3. *Fluid retention*
Reduced renal perfusion and the elevation of the venous
pressure cause fluid retention. A low serum albumin
secondary to nephrotic syndrome, protein-losing enteropathy
or hepatic dysfunction (all of which may complicate
pericardial constriction) reduces intravascular oncotic pressure
thereby exacerbating extravascular fluid accumulation.

Physical findings

1. *General appearance*
Evidence of weight loss, cachexia, chronic peripheral
oedema, ascites and jaundice (and other features of hepatic
dysfunction) are common. Cool extremities and peripheral
cyanosis may complicate the low cardiac output.

2. *Venous pressure*
A normal venous pressure virtually excludes a diagnosis of
constrictive pericarditis. Rarely does the venous pressure fall
with diuretic therapy. Marked elevation of the jugular venous
pressure is typical, and the dominant waves are negative with
deep and rapid 'x' and 'y' descents usually of equal
amplitude. Thickening of the pericardium prevents changes in
the intrathoracic pressure being transmitted to the venous
pressure. In severe constriction the venous pressure may
actually increase with inspiration (Kussmaul's sign).

3. *Arterial pulse*
A low systemic blood pressure and small pulse pressure
complicate the low cardiac output. Less than 50% of patients
exhibit arterial paradox which is seldom more than
15 mmHg. Inability to alter the stroke volume accounts for
the frequent compensatory tachycardia. An irregular pulse
due to atrial arrhythmias is present in 25% of cases and
accompanies atrial enlargement complicating long-standing
disease.

4. *Precordial impulses*
The apical impulse is impalpable in most patients but systolic
retraction of the cardiac apex may be perceived.

5. *Heart sounds*
S1 and S2 are normal, but occasionally A2 is premature due
to the reduction in LV stroke volume. Abrupt termination of
ventricular filling in early diastole causes an audible

pericardial 'knock' 60–120 ms after A2. This sound is similar in frequency but later in timing to a mitral opening snap, and higher in frequency and earlier in timing to a normal S3. Murmurs of mild mitral or tricuspid regurgitation may be present.

6. *Hepatic enlargement*
Elevated right-sided pressures cause hepatic enlargement and ascites. Chronic venous hypertension may result in cirrhosis which can be mistaken for a primary hepatic abnormality.

7. *Peripheral oedema and ascites*
Ascites occurs early in patients with pericardial constriction, and is more marked than lower limb oedema.
Hypoalbuminaemia may contribute to the extravascular fluid loss.

Investigations

1. *Blood tests*
Normochromic normocytic anaemia is seen in long-standing disease. Abnormalities of liver function include elevated bilirubin, alkaline phosphatase and gamma globulin, together with increased hepatic enzymes, low serum albumin, and depleted clotting factors (prolonged PT and KCT).
Proteinuria and protein loss from the gut may be marked and are reversible following successful pericardial resection.

2. *Electrocardiogram*
The ECG is rarely normal in pericardial constriction. Approximately 25% of patients are in atrial fibrillation (or flutter). Prolonged atrial depolarisation (pseudo P mitrale) occurs in 25% of patients. The insulation effect of the pericardial thickening and fibrosis cause a low voltage ECG with a mean QRS amplitude of 10 mm or less in half the patients. Repolarisation abnormalities (widespread T wave flattening or inversion) is almost universal. Significant Q waves occur in 5–10% of cases and may cause diagnostic confusion.

3. *Chest radiograph*
Pericardial constriction is one of the cardiac conditions in which the heart does not become enlarged. In uncomplicated constriction the heart size is normal although there may be left atrial prominence and distension of the superior vena cava. An increase in the cardiothoracic ratio usually indicates an additional pericardial effusion (see effusive-constrictive pericarditis). Pericardial calcification is present in 30–60% of patients, and is seen most readily on the left lateral radiograph running along the atrioventricular groove, the left heart border, and the anterior and diaphragmatic aspects of

the right ventricle. Pericardial calcification is not specific for tuberculous pericarditis, nor does it necessarily imply constriction.

4. *M-mode and cross-sectional echocardiography*
Pericardial thickening may be identified on both M-mode and cross sectional echocardiography, but the presence of a thickened pericardium does not necessarily indicate constriction; occasional patients with constriction have a normal pericardial appearance on echocardiography. Increased echodensity and parallel motion of the two pericardial layers implies pericardial adherence. Rapid LV dimension increase in early diastole is followed by sudden cessation of movement coincident with the pericardial knock. Septal movement may be paradoxical.

5. *Haemodynamics*
Cardiac catheterisation is needed to document the abnormal haemodynamics and *may* help differentiate constrictive pericarditis from restrictive cardiomyopathy. Simultaneous left and right heart catheterisation is undertaken as described in Chapter 20.

The following features are typical of pericardial constriction:
a. Elevated RA pressure with deep 'x' and 'y' descents
b. Respiratory changes in RA pressure are damped or absent
c. RA pressure may increase on inspiration
d. PACWP, RV and LV pressures all fall with inspiration
e. Moderate elevation in PA pressure (35–40 mm systolic)
f. Indices of LV systolic function (V_{CF}, V_{MAX}, ejection fraction) normal until late in the disease
g. Cardiac output maintained in low normal range by increased heart rate
h. Rapid early diastolic filling is seen as a 'dip' in the ventricular pressure trace, followed by a 'plateau' when late diastolic filling is limited by the constrictive process
i. LV and RV end diastolic pressures are *equal*, and rarely do the mean atrial pressures differ by more than 5 mmHg
j. Mild arterial paradox (<15 mmHg) is present in <50% of patients.

6. *Cineangiography*
Left ventricular cineangiography demonstrates normal dimensions and systolic function. Straightening of the right heart border may be visualised after a superior vena caval injection, and pericardial thickening may be implied from the increased distance between the LV cavity and the limit of the cardiac silhouette. However, echocardiography (or thoracic CT) is superior for this purpose.

EFFUSIVE-CONSTRICTIVE PERICARDITIS

This term refers to patients who have a pericardial effusion in addition to a thickened and fibrotic pericardium. Clinical and haemodynamic features are those of pericardial tamponade and are not relieved by pericardial aspiration. Pericardial resection is required in these patients.

OCCULT PERICARDITIS

A subgroup of patients have been described who present with atypical chest pain, fatigue, and non-specific repolarisation abnormalities on their ECG and develop abnormal haemodynamics following volume loading. Intracardiac pressures are normal in the resting state, but after infusion of one litre of normal saline over 5–10 minutes all the haemodynamic characteristics of pericardial constriction are seen. Pericardial resection may be beneficial in these cases.

Differential diagnosis

1. *Restrictive cardiomyopathy* (see Ch. 6)
   Differentiation between constrictive pericarditis and restrictive cardiomyopathy cannot always be made with certainty, particularly as a 'myocardial' element is seen in longstanding pericardial constriction. In view of the very poor prognosis in restrictive cardiomyopathy (and in unrelieved pericardial constriction), a patient should be subjected to exploratory thoracotomy if there is reasonable doubt as to the diagnosis.
   The following features of restrictive cardiomyopathy may help to distinguish it from pericardial constriction:
   a. Elevation in PA pressure may be marked (systolic >60 mmHg)
   b. LVEDP may exceed RVEDP by 5 mmHg or more particularly on exertion
   c. LV dimensions may be reduced due to LV hypertrophy
   d. Pericardial calcification is absent in restrictive cardiomyopathy
   e. Endomyocardial biopsy is diagnostic in some cases of restrictive cardiomyopathy (e.g. amyloid).
   NB: A 'dip and plateau' pattern can occur with either condition.
2. *Cardiac tamponade*
   With the advent of echocardiography, cardiac tamponade can be rapidly diagnosed with certainty and non-invasively.

Clinical signs that differentiate cardiac tamponade include:
a. Elevated venous pressure with a dominant 'x' descent, and reduced or absent 'y' descent
b. Venous pressure falls on inspiration
c. Marked arterial paradox.

Management

Surgical resection of the diseased pericardium is the treatment of choice for constrictive pericarditis. Patients with pericardial constriction frequently present late in the course of their disease at which time further delay in surgical intervention is inappropriate. Delay increases the operative risk and reduces the likelihood of a satisfactory haemodynamic result because of irreversible myocardial dysfunction.

Pericardial stripping is achieved via a left thoracotomy or median sternotomy. Some surgeons advocate cardiopulmonary bypass which may reduce the operative risk and allow a more radical procedure to be undertaken but this is usually unnecesary. Thickened pericardium is removed from both ventricles up to and including the atrioventricular groove, taking care to preserve the phrenic nerves and the coronary arteries. In end-stage disease difficulty may be encountered in finding a tissue plane between the thickened pericardium and the underlying epicardium. Cross-hatching the remaining pericardium may be helpful. Specimens of pericardium are sent to the laboratory for microscopy and culture (including AAFB). If tuberculosis is confirmed the patient should receive antituberculous chemotherapy as per one of the standard regimens for 6–12 months. The operative mortality for pericardectomy is approximately 5%.

Haemodynamic improvement may not occur for weeks or months and most patients will require diuretics for some time. Symptomatic benefit occurs in 75% of patients, although atrial arrhythmias usually persist despite successful surgery.

14. PULMONARY EMBOLISM

A spectrum of conditions resulting from obstruction of one or more pulmonary arteries usually by thrombus arising from the lower limbs, pelvic veins, or rarely the upper limbs or right atrium. Presentation is variable ranging from the asymptomatic to sudden death. Pulmonary embolism is frequently undiagnosed which is unfortunate because appropriate treatment leads to a reduction in morbidity and mortality. It is useful to consider pulmonary embolism as minor, acute massive, subacute massive and chronic because the presentation, treatment and prognosis of each category differs.

AETIOLOGY

Venous thrombosis is related to:
1. Changes in the vessel wall (e.g. trauma)
2. Changes in blood flow (e.g. stasis)
3. Changes in the blood (e.g. increased platelet adhesiveness, aggregation etc.).

RISK FACTORS

1. Bed rest
2. Increasing age
3. Surgery (especially pelvis, abdomen and obstetric)
4. Heart disease including acute myocardial infarction
5. Oestrogens (>50 μg/day)
6. Obesity
7. Nephrotic syndrome
8. Chronic airflow obstruction
9. Previous deep vein thrombosis or thrombophlebitis
10. Occult carcinoma
11. Pregnancy
12. Trauma

MINOR PULMONARY EMBOLISM

Minor pulmonary embolism causes no haemodynamic disturbance and complications are rare. However, 30–50% of patients who experience major embolism have previously sustained minor emboli. Minor emboli usually lyse spontaneously and pulmonary infarction is uncommon (10–15%). As the clinical diagnosis of all forms of pulmonary embolism is unreliable (approximately 40% correct), and the inappropriate use of anticoagulants and thrombolytic agents is potentially hazardous, it is important to confirm the clinical suspicion with certainty by means of appropriate investigations.

Symptoms

1. Pleuritic chest pain (40%)
2. Cough (50%) ± haemoptysis (40%)
3. Breathlessness/hyperventilation
4. From deep vein thrombosis (e.g. painful swollen leg) (80%)

Physical signs

1. Tachypnoea (80%)
2. Fever (40%)
3. Chest signs
   pleural rub (10–20%)
   crackles
   reduced air entry (pleural effusion)
   bronchial breathing (consolidation)
4. Source of emboli (e.g. DVT)

Investigations

1. *Chest radiograph*
   Pulmonary emboli tend to affect the lower lobes due to preferential blood flow to these areas (except in recumbent patients and those with mitral valve disease).

   Features
   a. Normal (>50%)
   b. Elevated hemidiaphragm
   c. Pulmonary oligaemia (uncommon)
   d. Enlarged hilar arteries
   e. Tapering of occluded vessel
   f. 'Plate' (linear) atelectasis
   g. Pleural effusion/haemorrhage usually indicates infarction
   h. Consolidation

2. *Electrocardiography*

Normal or non-specific repolarisation changes. Minor frontal plane axis shift to the right (compared with previous records if available). No correlation with resolution.

3. *Arterial blood gases*

Reduced PaO_2, reduced $PaCO_2$ (increased A-a gradient), respiratory alkalosis. PaO_2 (>9.0 kPa) in 10% of patients.

4. *Enzymes*

Elevated lactate dehydrogenase (LDH) with a normal aspartate aminotransferase (AAT). Unreliable.

5. *Pulmonary scintigraphy*

a. *Perfusion* (Q)

Following intravenous injection of ^{99m}Tc macroaggregated albumin, minor pulmonary emboli are seen as multiple focal perfusion defects which are segmental or wedge-shaped and frequently situated on the pleural surface of the lung. Single lesions which are not segmental or lobar in distribution or are circular in shape are less specific and may accompany other forms of respiratory or cardiac disease (e.g. chronic airflow obstruction or chronic pulmonary oedema). Perfusion scanning is a very sensitive test and a normal scan taken with multiple views virtually excludes a pulmonary embolism; a perfusion scan is particularly helpful in the presence of a normal chest radiograph when there are few (if any) false negatives.

b. *Ventilation-perfusion* (V/Q)

Combination of perfusion (^{99m}Tc) and ventilation (^{81}Kr or ^{133}Xe) allows separation of matched ventilation and perfusion defects (e.g. chronic airflow obstruction, pulmonary fibrosis etc.), from V/Q mismatch (ventilated but unperfused areas of lung) typical of pulmonary embolism. Perfusion scans in patients who have previously experienced pulmonary emboli lack specificity as scans may remain abnormal for months or years after the initial event.

6. *Pulmonary arteriography*

Although this invasive technique requires a catheterisation laboratory and the necessary expertise, the high sensitivity and specificity is associated with a low morbidity and mortality in experienced hands. In minor embolism arteriography is reserved for cases in whom the diagnosis is uncertain and pulmonary embolism needs excluding in the presence of a normal chest radiograph and abnormal perfusion scan (see massive pulmonary embolism for details of method).

7. *Investigation of source of emboli*

The majority of pulmonary emboli (80%) arise in the lower

limbs. Clinical diagnosis of deep venous thrombosis is incorrect in at least 50% of cases. Lower limb veins can be visualised by pedal venography up to the level of the inguinal ligament. Satisfactory demonstration of thrombus in the pelvic veins is difficult but can usually be achieved by a combination of pedal venograms and an inferior vena cavagram. If the source of emboli remains obscure, cross-sectional echocardiography may demonstrate thrombus within the right atrium or ventricle, or an abnormality of the tricuspid valve (e.g. vegetations).

Differential diagnosis

1. Respiratory infection
2. Pleurisy
3. Chest wall pain
4. Hyperventilation syndrome

Treatment

Anticoagulation is the mainstay of treatment.
1. *Heparin*
   Heparin 10 000 units by intravenous bolus, followed by 40 000 units per day by continuous infusion adjusted to maintain the kaolin cephalin time (KCT) at ×2–3 control value. Continue heparin until warfarin therapeutic.
2. *Warfarin*
   Commence warfarin orally on day one. Load with 10 mg on each day for three days, check the prothrombin time on day 4 and give an adequate dose of warfarin (usually 2–10 mg daily) to maintain the British Standard Prothrombin Ratio at 2.5–3.0. Patient should remain on warfarin for three months assuming the stimulus to thromboembolism (e.g. surgery) has been removed. Further minor emboli in patients who are adequately anticoagulated are rare.

ACUTE MASSIVE PULMONARY EMBOLISM

Pulmonary embolism involving 50% or more of the pulmonary arterial tree. In patients with pre-existing heart or lung disease lesser emboli may have the features of massive pulmonary embolism. Death results from a reduction in cardiac output as a consequence of acute right ventricular failure. Prompt diagnosis, investigation and treatment is mandatory.

Symptoms

1. Dizziness or syncope
2. Shock or circulatory arrest (usually asystolic) (30%)
3. Dyspnoea (80%), cough ± haemoptysis (20%)
4. Retrosternal chest pain indistinguishable from angina pectoris (30%) (cause uncertain ?RV ischaemia, ?pericardial distension)
5. Sudden death (60% of patients die within two hours)

Physical signs

1. *Shock*
   Sweating, oliguria, impaired cerebration and systemic hypotension. Patients with massive pulmonary embolism prefer to lie flat (contrast with acute myocardial infarction and pulmonary oedema) because the blood pressure falls on sitting upright
2. *Heart rate*
   Sinus tachycardia. Arrhythmias uncommon.
3. *Cyanosis*
   Peripheral: poor perfusion, low cardiac output.
   Central: V/Q mismatch due to mechanical obstruction or vasoconstriction (serotonin etc) and/or patent foramen ovale.
4. *Venous pressure*
   Elevated venous pressure (prominent 'a' wave).
5. *Heart sounds*
   Right-sided S3 and S4 (no accentuation of P2 as PA pressure rarely greater than 40–50 mm Hg).

Investigations

1. *Chest radiograph*
   a. Normal
   b. Oligaemia (>80%) plus compensatory hyperaemia (40%)
   c. Prominent main pulmonary arteries (50%)
   d. Acute pulmonary oedema
2. *Electrocardiogram*
   a. Normal (changes may be delayed and/or transient)
   b. Sinus tachycardia (± low voltage)
   c. Right atrial P wave
   d. Right-sided 'strain' RAD
   $\qquad\qquad\qquad$ RBBB
   $\qquad\qquad\qquad$ SI, QIII, T ↓ III
   $\qquad\qquad\qquad$ SI, QIII, T ↓ III, T ↓ $V_{1-3/4}$
   e. Left-sided changes (?due to pre-existing coronary disease)
   $\qquad$ T ↓ V_{4-6}

3. *Arterial blood gases*
   As for minor pulmonary embolism.
4. *Pulmonary arteriography*
   Right heart catheterisation from the right antecubital, subclavian or femoral vein. Pigtail or NIH (7F) catheter to right atrium, right ventricle and main PA. Measure pressures and PA oxygen saturation in addition to arterial saturation to calculate cardiac output (see Ch. 21). Pulmonary arteriogram recorded in AP projection using 0.5 ml/kg contrast medium (e.g. Isopaque) at 20 ml/s after a test injection. If test injection clears slowly (due to major proximal artery occlusion) give half the dose. In critically ill patients use non-ionic contrast medium (e.g. Niopam). Record arteriograms on cut-film (rather than cine) which is more suitable for analysing detail of the anatomy of the small pulmonary vessels. Typical cases show arterial cut-offs, intravascular filling defects, segmental hypoperfusion and delayed venous return to the affected areas. Additional views (e.g. selective or oblique) may be necessary to further define the anatomy. Pulmonary arteriography is the only suitable method for distinguishing recurrent embolism from fragmentation and distal migration for existing thrombus. Consider leaving the catheter insitu for regional thrombolytic therapy and follow-up arteriography 48 hours after the initial study.

Differential diagnosis

1. *Acute myocardial infarction*
   Chest pain ± orthopnoea or pulmonary oedema. ECG and cardiac enzymes.
2. *Pericardial tamponade*
   Systemic hypotension and arterial paradox. Cross-sectional echocardiography.
3. *Aortic dissection*
   Check peripheral pulses and for signs of aortic regurgitation. Chest radiograph, cross-sectional echocardiography, CT scan and aortography.
4. *Respiratory failure*
   Hyperventilation, previous chronic airflow obstruction. Elevated $PaCO_2$.
5. *Haemorrhage*
   Evident blood loss, pale and sweaty, low venous pressure.
6. *Gram negative septicaemia*
   Fever (not always), vasodilatation and low venous pressure.
7. *Tension pneumothorax*
   Reduced air entry, mediastinal shift. Chest radiography.

Treatment

1. *Resuscitation* (see also Ch. 20)
   a. Maintain airway
   b. Administer sodium bicarbonate to correct metabolic acidosis
   c. Maintain adequate right ventricular 'preload' with colloid
   d. Intermittent positive pressure ventilation if necessary (high FIO_2 to maintain $PaO_2 > 10.0$ kPa if possible)
   e. External cardiac massage (may break-up and disperse thrombi in addition to maintaining tissue perfusion)
   f. Circulatory support
      Beta agonists (e.g. Isoprenaline $0.02-0.1$ $\mu g/kg/min$ or salbutamol 0.5 $\mu g/kg/min$) may reduce right ventricular impedance by lowering pulmonary vascular resistance. Renal doses of dopamine ($2-5$ $\mu g/kg/min$) may also be required.
   g. Partial femoro-femoral bypass (if available).
2. *Medical therapy*
   a. Anticoagulation
      ?Heparin bolus 100 000 units (antiserotonin effect) — beneficial effect unproven in man. Standard regimen as for minor embolism.
   b Fibrinolysis
      Streptokinase (infused into the pulmonary artery), 250 000 units as a bolus followed by 100 000 units per hour for 48 hours and repeat pulmonary arteriogram. Monitor thrombin time (TT) to maintain at $\times 2-4$ normal (laboratory monitoring is not essential). Contraindications to thrombolytic therapy include bleeding diathesis, peptic ulceration, early postoperative period (?), recent diagnostic procedures (e.g. lumbar puncture), previous streptokinase (cover with steroids), cerebrovascular haemorrhage and severe systemic hypertension.
      NB: Insert all lines (CVP, arterial etc.) prior to administration of thrombolytic agents in order to avoid local bleeding complications. Take blood specimens from indwelling line rather than from needle stick. Bleeding complications (most of which are minor) occur in $35-75\%$ of patients.
3. *Surgical intervention*
   Pulmonary embolectomy using cardiopulmonary bypass in experienced hands has a mortality of $20-25\%$ in patients that have survived two hours. Mortality increases dramatically (approximately 66%) if embolectomy is carried out following cardiac arrest, due mainly to anoxic cerebral damage. There is no place for the formerly advocated procedures of

pulmonary embolectomy without cardiopulmonary bypass (e.g. Trendelenburg operation with outflow occlusion, or modified Trendelenburg with inflow occlusion) as the mortality is unacceptable (80%). An alternative approach in centres without facilities for cardiopulmonary bypass is transfemoral removal of pulmonary emboli in which a large 'bell-mouthed' suction catheter is introduced via the right femoral artery and the emboli are sucked out of the pulmonary circulation under fluoroscopic control; early reports using this technique are encouraging.

Choice of treatment in acute massive pulmonary embolism

Having confirmed the clinical diagnosis, the choice of treatment lies between thrombolysis or pulmonary embolectomy using cardiopulmonary bypass. Dissolution of thrombus occurs more rapidly with thrombolysis followed by heparin when compared with heparin alone, but the long-term results are similar. Streptokinase is less expensive than urokinase and if all patients are covered with a single dose of corticosteroid (hydrocortisone sodium succinate 100 mg IV), allergic reactions are limited to the occasional fever; the efficacy of the two lytic agents is similar. If the expertise is available, pulmonary embolectomy is the treatment of choice for patients who are in cardiogenic shock or if thrombolysis is contraindicated. A meaningful comparison between medical and surgical treatment is impossible on available data. A suggested protocol for the treatment of acute massive pulmonary embolism is shown in Figure 14.1.

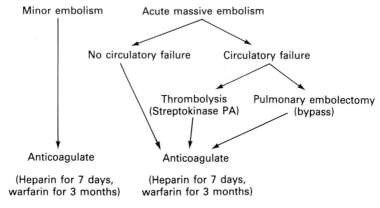

Fig. 14.1 Treatment of acute massive pulmonary embolism

SUBACUTE MASSIVE PULMONARY EMBOLISM

A small subgroup of patients presenting late (>14 days) in whom acute massive pulmonary embolism has been inadequately treated. Large areas (>50%) of the pulmonary arterial tree are occluded by adherent and organized emboli which respond poorly to anticoagulation, late thrombolysis or embolectomy. The high mortality in these patients emphasizes the importance of early and aggressive treatment of massive pulmonary embolism.

CHRONIC THROMBOEMBOLIC PULMONARY HYPERTENSION

Long-term sequelae following acute pulmonary embolism occur in less than 5% of patients; in particular, chronic thromboembolic pulmonary hypertension is rarely seen.

Chronic thromboembolic pulmonary hypertension is an uncommon condition which presents insidiously and may be indistinguishable from primary pulmonary hypertension (see Ch. 15). Progressive breathlessness, fatigue, anorexia and lower limb oedema is associated wtih atypical chest pain and episodes of dizziness or syncope. Discrete episodes suggestive of thromboembolism are rarely a feature of the clinical history.

Physical findings include pulmonary hypertension, right heart failure and fluid retention. Chest radiography reveals dilatation of the proximal pulmonary arteries and relative oligaemia ('pruning') of the peripheral pulmonary vessels.

Most authorities advocate long-term anticoagulation in these patients, but evidence that this approach alters prognosis is anecdotal. Where repeated lower limb thromboembolism has been documented, inferior vena caval plication or insertion of an umbrella may have a role in the prevention of recurrence.

15. PULMONARY HYPERTENSION

PRIMARY PULMONARY HYPERTENSION

Primary pulmonary hypertension (PPH) is a diagnosis of exclusion based on the findings of clinical, electrocardiographic and radiographic evidence of idiopathic pulmonary arterial hypertension confirmed by haemodynamic studies. Cardiac catheterisation reveals a variable elevation in pulmonary artery pressure, which in severe cases is suprasystemic, a normal pulmonary arterial wedge pressure, a normal or reduced cardiac output, and an elevated pulmonary vascular resistance. Because of the poor prognostic implications of the condition, it is crucial to exclude other causes of 'secondary' pulmonary hypertension which may be more amenable to treatment. These include any cause of an elevated left atrial pressure (e.g. mitral stenosis, left ventricular disease), pulmonary veno-occlusive disease, pulmonary hypertension secondary to lung disease (cor pulmonale, see p. 227), and pulmonary hypertension complicating high pulmonary blood flow (e.g. congenital heart disease, arteriovenous malformations).

Aetiology

Although the cause of PPH is unclear, a number of factors may be important in the development of the condition. These include:

1. *Appetite suppressants*
   In the late 1960s a proportion of patients taking an amphetamine-like appetite suppressant called Aminorex developed a clinical syndrome indistinguishable from PPH with similar pathological features. The fact that only a small percentage of these patients developed the condition suggests a predisposition or idiosyncracy. Reversal of the haemodynamic abnormalities was not uncommon. A cause and effect relationship between Aminorex and pulmonary hypertension has not been confirmed in any animal model. Other drugs that have been implicated in the development of the disease include phenformin, chloramphenicol and sulphonamides.

2. *Alkaloids*

   Toxic hepatic metabolites of the pyrrolizidine alkaloid monocrotaline cause pulmonary hypertension in the rat, dog and monkey. This alkaloid is present in the seeds of the shrub Crotalaria spectabilis; and another alkaloid, fulvine, occurs in C. fulva. Monocrotaline is a constituent of 'bush tea' and has also been implicated in the genesis of veno-occlusive disease of the liver.

3. *Autoimmune disease*

   Pulmonary hypertension may be the first manifestation of autoimmune disease (e.g. systemic lupus erythematosus). Patients with PPH have a higher than expected incidence of positive antinuclear antibodies and Raynaud's phenomenon. Pulmonary hypertension may also be a feature of scleroderma or CREST syndrome and polyarteritis nodosum.

4. *Thromboembolic disease*

   A proportion of patients thought on clinical grounds to have PPH are found to have thromboemboli at post mortem. Although the two conditions can coexist, the pathological changes in PPH are characteristic and can be differentiated from thromboembolic disease. In situ thrombosis may occur and the role of pulmonary arteriolar spasm in the pathogenesis of PPH remains to be defined.

5. *Altitude*

   PPH is seen more frequently in patients living at altitude and may improve on returning to sea level.

6. *Familial studies*

   Familial clustering of cases is well described usually with autosomal dominant inheritance. PPH in twins has also been reported.

7. *Pregnancy*

   Examples of PPH presenting during or shortly after pregnancy have been well documented. A proportion of these cases may represent pulmonary hypertension secondary to thromboembolism or amniotic fluid embolism, but the association of PPH and pregnancy is undoubtedly real. PPH may also occur with (or be exacerbated by) oral contraceptives.

8. *Portal hypertension*

   Cirrhosis of the liver complicated by portal hypertension may be associated with pulmonary hypertension. Although some of these cases are thromboembolic in origin the pathological changes seen in the lung are usually identical to those seen in PPH.

9. *Infestation*
   PPH is seen more commonly in areas where filariasis (due to Wucheria Bancrofti) is endemic.
10. *Congenital defect*
    Persistence of the foetal pattern of pulmonary artery histology may be responsible for the occurrence of PPH in infants and young children.

Pathology

The classic pathological feature of PPH is plexogenic pulmonary arteriopathy. Although typical of PPH, the 'plexogenic' lesion may also be seen in pulmonary hypertension complicating congenital heart disease and hepatic cirrhosis. Pathological changes are patchy in distribution and may vary in severity throughout the parenchyma of the lung.
They include:

1. Atherosclerosis in the large pulmonary arteries
2. Concentric intimal thickening and fibrosis (so-called 'onionskin' appearance)
3. Medial hypertrophy of muscular pulmonary arteries and muscularisation of the pulmonary arterioles
4. Fibrinoid necrosis of the media secondary to a necrotising vasculitis
5. 'Plexiform' lesions: dilated branches of muscular arteries that resemble veins, occurring as a result of intimal proliferation and medial degeneration.

The severity of the arteriopathy does not relate to the elevation in pulmonary arterial pressure or pulmonary vascular resistance, nor to the prognosis in a particular patient. It has been suggested therefore that a 'vasospastic' component may be partially responsible for the haemodynamic derangement. In thromboembolic disease 'plexogenic' lesions are absent, and thromboemboli are found in various stages of organisation.

Clinical features

Patients with PPH become symptomatic late in the course of their illness such that by the time the diagnosis is made the signs of pulmonary hypertension are severe and most patients die within 2–3 years. The disease may occur at any age, but it is most common in young adults with females affected more frequently than males (3–4:1). In occasional patients PPH runs a protracted course and very rarely the hypertension has been seen to regress.

Symptoms

The symptoms are those of pulmonary hypertension, and are not specific for PPH.

1. *Dyspnoea*
   Exertional dyspnoea, lethargy and fatigue are the most common symptoms and occur as a result of a low cardiac output which does not increase appropriately with exercise. Hyperventilation at rest may be striking.

2. *Chest pain*
   Chest pain in patients with PPH is usually non-specific but right ventricular ischaemia can cause typical angina. Pleurisy may complicate pulmonary emboli which arise secondary to the low forward flow or from thrombus formation in the dilated right heart.

3. *Dizziness and syncope*
   A failure to increase cardiac output on exertion causes dizziness and syncope. Sudden death is not uncommon. Over enthusiastic use of vasodilators or diuretics results in similar symptoms.

4. *Cough*
   A non-productive cough may be troublesome. Major haemoptysis is uncommon. Direct pressure from an enlarged left pulmonary artery may compress the recurrent laryngeal nerve and cause hoarseness of the voice.

5. *Palpitations*
   Atrial and ventricular premature beats, atrial fibrillation, and ventricular tachycardia complicate the elevated right-sided pressures.

6. *Fluid retention*
   Late in the course of the illness the falling cardiac output causes secondary hyperaldosteronism which results in fluid retention and weight gain.

Physical signs

1. *Low cardiac output*
   In severe pulmonary hypertension, poor peripheral perfusion and peripheral cyanosis is associated with a small volume pulse and sinus tachycardia. Central cyanosis is uncommon.

2. *Venous pressure*
   Pulmonary arterial hypertension is reflected in the prominent 'a' wave in the venous pressure. A low cardiac output and fluid retention is associated with an elevated venous pressure and tricuspid regurgitation causes a systolic ('cv') wave to be present.

3. *Precordial impulses*

Right ventricular hypertrophy causes a sustained left parasternal impulse. Dilatation of the main pulmonary artery and pulmonary valve closure (P2) results in a visible and palpable pulsation in the second left intercostal space.

4. *Heart sounds and murmurs*

S1 is normal. S2 is narrowly split with an accentuated pulmonary component. A right atrial fourth sound is not uncommon, and a systolic ejection click (with or without the early diastolic murmur of pulmonary regurgitation) can be frequently heard in the pulmonary area due to pulmonary arterial dilatation. With dilatation of the tricuspid annulus a pansystolic murmur (which increases on inspiration) indicates tricuspid regurgitation with an additional S3 when the regurgitation is severe.

5. *Other features*

Right heart failure with lower limb oedema, hepatic enlargement and ascites is seen late in the illness.

Investigations

1. *Chest radiograph*

At the time of presentation, the cardiothoracic ratio is usually normal. On the PA projection, the main pulmonary artery is dilated and appears larger than the aortic knuckle. The proximal left and right pulmonary arteries are also enlarged but there is rapid tapering of the more distal vessels such that the peripheral lung fields appear oligaemic (so called 'pruning'). With increasing tricuspid regurgitation, the right atrium dilates and may become very large causing the cardiothoracic ratio to increase.

2. *Electrocardiography*

The ECG is relatively insensitive at detecting right ventricular hypertrophy secondary to PPH. Typical features include right axis deviation (mean QRS axis $+120°$ or greater in adults), a dominant R wave in V_1, an R wave of >0.9 mV in V_1 in adults, a qR or an rSR' pattern in V_1, and associated right atrial dilatation and hypertrophy (P 'pulmonale' i.e. P wave >0.2 mV in lead II). Other causes of a dominant R wave in V_1 are true posterior infarction, RBBB, Wolff-Parkinson-White syndrome (with left bypass tract) and dextrocardia. Repolarisation abnormalities (downsloping or horizontal ST depression) may be striking in the right precordial leads.

3. *M-mode and cross-sectional echocardiography*

Patients with PPH have the features of pulmonary hypertension on M-mode and cross-sectional echocardiography. An accurate assessment of right ventricular hypertrophy is difficult to obtain in adults, as much of the right ventricle lies beneath the sternum and is not accessible to the M-mode technique. In occasional patients pulmonary hypertension causes asymmetric septal hypertrophy. Right ventricular dilatation may be present and reversed septal motion accompanies tricuspid regurgitation. Mid-systolic closure or notching of the pulmonary valve is a valuable sign of pulmonary arterial hypertension. Cross-sectional echocardiography frequently reveals dilatation of the pulmonary artery, which may also occur in situations of high flow (e.g. ASD). Abnormalities of the pulmonary valve may also be visualised by cross-sectional echocardiography. Left ventricular function and the mitral valve appear normal, thus excluding left-sided disease.

4. *Pulmonary scintigraphy*
Pulmonary perfusion scans using ^{99m}Tc human albumin microspheres are either normal, or show non-specific subsegmental defects. Most patients with thromboembolic pulmonary hypertension exhibit larger segmental defects on scintigraphy. Perfusion scanning may be hazardous in these patients due to obstruction of small pulmonary vessels by microspheres.

5. *Pulmonary function tests*
A low K_{co} may occur, but pulmonary function tests are usually unremarkable. Changes in arterial blood gases are indistinguishable from those of pulmonary embolism, namely a low PCO_2 secondary to hyperventilation which results in a respiratory alkalosis, a normal or slightly reduced PaO_2, and an increased A-a gradient.

6. *Cardiac catheterisation and pulmonary arteriography*
The haemodynamic features of PPH are non-specific, but cardiac catheterisation can exclude secondary causes of pulmonary hypertension. Catheterisation of the right heart is achieved using a standard technique (Ch. 20), and a full left and right-sided saturation run is taken to exclude a left to right shunt as a cause of the pulmonary hypertension. Occasionally in severe PPH, arterial desaturation will be found as a consequence of right to left shunting through a patent foramen ovale. Every attempt should be made to record a high quality pulmonary arterial wedge pressure, but this may be technically difficult. A balloon flotation (Swan-Ganz) catheter may pass more readily to the wedge position.

Pulmonary arteriography may be hazardous if the pulmonary hypertension is severe (>100 mmHg), and selective arteriography or a magnification pulmonary wedge arteriogram may be preferable. Use of a non-ionic contrast agent (e.g. Niopam) reduces the load on the right ventricle. Arteriography demonstrates dilated proximal pulmonary arteries, which taper rapidly giving a 'cork-screw' appearance. A paucity of small peripheral vessels on the late arterial phase is apparent, and venous filling is delayed. Arterial 'cut-offs' and filling defects (typical of thromboemboli) are absent.

The effect of breathing 100% oxygen for 15 minutes, followed by the acute administration of various vasodilators is undertaken. None of these agents is specific for the pulmonary circulation, therefore changes in pulmonary and systemic pressures, pulmonary and systemic vascular resistances and cardiac output must all be recorded, together with associated symptomatic changes.

7. *Other tests*
Hypoxia in PPH is rarely severe enough to cause polycythaemia. Various abnormalities of clotting and thrombolysis have been described in association with PPH.

Treatment

The assessment of treatment in patients with PPH is complicated by a number of factors. The natural history of PPH in an individual patient is unknown. Spontaneous variations in subjective exercise tolerance are not uncommon, and although the overall prognosis is poor, occasional regression in cases of pulmonary hypertension has been documented.

In acute studies, changes in pulmonary arterial pressure and pulmonary vascular resistance may not concur due to secondary effects on cardiac output. Furthermore, the variability in pulmonary arterial pressure seen from hour to hour in an individual patient, particularly in those with an elevated pulmonary vascular resistance, may make the correct interpretation of the haemodynamic effects of drugs difficult or impossible.

1. *Vasodilators*
Various drugs have been tried including beta agonists, alpha blockers, calcium channel blockers, smooth muscle relaxants and prostaglandins. An intravenous or oral trial of any one of these agents should be carried out with extreme caution (preferably with monitoring in an ICU environment) because profound changes in systemic vascular resistance may precipitate systemic hypotension.

Patients with PPH present late in the course of their illness by which time the elevation in pulmonary vascular resistance is fixed, and the haemodynamic improvement brought about by drugs is minimal.

Criteria for the beneficial of a drug should include:
a. 20% reduction in PVR, and
b. Cardiac output increased or unchanged

    c. PA pressure is decreased or unchanged, and

    d. Systemic blood pressure unchanged, or reduced such that the patient does not experience side effects.

    Oral therapy is unlikely to be effective in a patient who has shown no haemodynamic improvement with an intravenous trial of the same agent. No drug has yet been shown to alter prognosis.

2. *Anticoagulants*

    Oral anticoagulation has been advocated on the basis that many patients dying of PPH are found to have small numbers of thrombosed arterioles at post-mortem together with the fact that PPH and thromboembolic pulmonary hypertension are difficult to differentiate clinically. An improvement in prognosis is difficult to prove and most authorities reserve anticoagulants for patients with thromboembolic pulmonary hypertension.

3. *Oxygen*

    Continuous low-flow oxygen may result in some symptomatic improvement in patients who are hypoxic (PaO_2, <8 kPa) when breathing air. The efficacy of oxygen in PPH is unproven.

4. *Heart-lung transplantation*

    With increasing experience, the technique of combined heart and lung transplantation may become a reasonable therapeutic option for patients with PPH and other forms of pulmonary hypertension.

COR PULMONALE

Cor pulmonale can be defined as right ventricular dysfunction secondary to pulmonary disease. Acute cor pulmonale is limited to pulmonary embolism (see Ch. 14); chronic cor pulmonale is caused by diseases affecting ventilation (either mechanical, or the neural control of ventilation), gas exchange, or the pulmonary vascular bed (Table 15.1). By definition, cor pulmonale excludes abnormalities of right ventricular function secondary to left-sided disease (e.g. mitral valve disease, ischaemic heart disease, cardiomyopathy); however there is evidence to suggest that left ventricular function is abnormal in some patients with cor pulmonale.

    The pulmonary circulation is a low resistance circuit with considerable reserve. Alterations in ventilation-perfusion relationships, and the ability to 'recruit' pulmonary vessels allows an increase in pulmonary blood flow without a significant change in pressure. In patients with mild pulmonary disease (e.g. chronic airflow obstruction), haemodynamics may be normal at rest, but become abnormal with exercise or during sleep (see p. 231).

Table 15.1 Causes of chronic cor pulmonale

1. Chronic airflow obstruction
    chronic obstructive bronchitis
    bronchial asthma
    emphysema

2. Chronic pulmonary infection
    cystic fibrosis
    bronchiectasis

3. Restrictive lung disease
    fibrosing alveolitis
    pulmonary fibrosis
    pleural fibrosis

4. Disorders of the thoracic cage
    kyphosis
    scoliosis
    post-surgical (e.g. thoracoplasty)

5. Upper airway obstruction
    tracheal stenosis
    tonsils and adenoids (children)
    sleep-apnoea syndrome

6. Abnormalities of respiratory control
    idiopathic hypoventilation syndrome
    obesity-hypoventilation syndrome
    cerebrovascular disease

Thus, the normal adaptive responses to increased pulmonary flow are impaired. Arterial hypoxaemia and pulmonary hypertension (intermittent or continuous) are pathognomonic of cor pulmonale.

Mechanisms of cor pulmonale

The mechanisms responsible for the development of pulmonary hypertension in a patient with pulmonary disease are unclear. A number of factors are probably important:

1. *Restriction of the pulmonary vascular bed*
    Patients with repeated thromboemboli develop pulmonary hypertension secondary to occlusion of pulmonary vessels, and a reduction in the number of vessels is the mechanism of pulmonary hypertension following extensive lung resection. A similar pattern may be observed in schistosomiasis, filariasis and sickle cell disease. However, pulmonary hypertension is an infrequent complication of emphysema in which pulmonary vessels are destroyed, and in experimental studies two thirds of the pulmonary vascular bed can be obliterated without any significant increase in pulmonary artery pressure.

2. *Constriction of pulmonary vessels*
    Arterial hypoxia results from alveolar hypoventilation, due either to a failure in ventilatory drive or from ventilation-perfusion abnormalities. Pulmonary artery pressure is related to PaO_2 (and SaO_2). Hypoxaemia leads to pulmonary hypertension by causing vasoconstriction of pulmonary

arterioles, either by the direct action of hypoxia on arterial smooth muscle, or via vasoactive substances (e.g. histamine) augmented by endogenous catecholamine release.

Hypercapnia and acidosis may exacerbate the elevation in pulmonary arterial pressure but there is little evidence to suggest that an elevated $PaCO_2$ or acidosis per se (without hypoxaemia) cause pulmonary hypertension. Chronic hypoxic vasoconstriction results in intimal proliferation and medial hypertrophy in the pulmonary arterioles. Thus, labile pulmonary hypertension becomes fixed due to a reduction in cross-sectional area of the vascular lumen and an inability to adapt to changes in pulmonary blood flow.

3. *Blood viscosity*
   Chronic hypoxia causes renal release of erythropoetin which leads to secondary polycythaemia. An elevated blood viscosity increases pulmonary vascular resistance and forward flow is reduced still further.

4. *Pulmonary blood flow*
   An increase in pulmonary blood flow (e.g. in intracardiac shunts) causes intimal proliferation and medial hypertrophy within pulmonary arterioles. This may be a factor in the development of pulmonary hypertension when the pulmonary vascular bed has been compromised due to (1) or (2) above and blood flow is increased in the remaining areas of lung.

Symptoms

Chronic airflow obstruction is the most common cause of cor pulmonale. An episode of cor pulmonale is often precipitated by a deterioration in respiratory function complicating a lower respiratory tract infection. Chronic bronchitis and emphysema frequently coexist but it is useful to classify patients (Table 15.2) into those with predominant bronchitis (so called 'blue bloaters') and those with emphysema ('pink puffers') because

Table 15.2 Clinical patterns of chronic airflow obstruction

Chronic obstructive bronchitis ('Blue bloaters')	Emphysema ('Pink puffers')
Sputum ++	Sputum ±
Breathless +	Breathless ++
Central cyanosis	Hyperinflation
Fluid retention	PaO_2 near normal
Cor pulmonale	$PaCO_2$ low
PaO_2 low (V/Q mismatch)	
$PaCO_2$ high (?central hypoventilation)	
Secondary polycythaemia	

NB: Correlation between clinical presentation and the underlying pathology (defined above) is poor the physiology and clinical features of each can be recognised and the treatment (and prognosis) of the two conditions differ.

Chronic obstructive bronchitis is characterised by chronic sputum production sufficient to cause expectoration and progressive breathlessness initially occurring on exertion and subsequently at rest. Symptoms of carbon dioxide retention may also be present including headache, lethargy, an inability to concentrate, confusion and tremor. Bouts of prolonged coughing can lead to loss of consciousness (cough syncope) as a result of vagal stimulation and reduced cerebral perfusion secondary to raised intracranial pressure.

Cor pulmonale is uncommon in association with restrictive lung disease probably because the PaO_2 at rest remains normal or near normal until late in the natural history of the condition. In pure emphysema (e.g. alpha$_1$ antitrypsin deficiency) cor pulmonale occurs late as a pre-terminal event.

Clinical features

1. *Pulmonary disease*

   Evidence of pulmonary disease includes tachypnoea, hyperinflation, use of accessory muscles and prolonged expiration. Auscultation of the lungs reveals inspiratory or expiratory crackles and expiratory wheezes depending on the nature of the pulmonary disease. Patients with pulmonary infection are frequently febrile and the signs of pneumonic consolidation may be obvious.

2. *Cyanosis*

   Central cyanosis is apparent when there is >5 g% reduced haemoglobin present in the arterial blood. Assuming a normal haemoglobin, this indicates that the PaO_2 will be <8 kPa (approximately) when breathing air. The low cardiac output associated with severe cor pulmonale results in peripheral cyanosis due to poor perfusion which may be compounded by vasodilatation secondary to CO_2 retention.

3. *Venous pressure*

   Fluid retention and right ventricular failure cause an elevated venous pressure and distended neck veins. Pulmonary hypertension is accompanied by a prominent 'a' wave and a systolic ('cv') wave occurs when dilatation of the right ventricle leads to tricuspid regurgitation. As a consequence of a raised venous pressure the liver is enlarged and tender, and chronic lower limb oedema may be striking often complicated by venous stasis and ulceration. Hyperinflated lungs and the depressed diaphragms may cause direct compression of the inferior vena cava and promote oedema of the legs.

4. *Auscultation of the heart*

   S1 is normal. Pulmonary hypertension causes accentuation of

P2 and a right sided S4. An S3 and a pansystolic murmur (both increasing on inspiration) indicate right ventricular failure and tricuspid regurgitation. Appreciation of these signs may be difficult because of extraneous noise from the lungs and the effects of hyperinflation on conduction of the heart sounds through the chest wall.

Investigations

1. *Blood tests*
   Routine testing should include a full blood count to document secondary polycythaemia and an elevated white count may indicate infection. A predominance of polymorphs favours pyogenic infection, whereas a lymphocytosis is compatible with viral infection or mycoplasma pneumoniae (in which case cold agglutinins are present in 70% of cases). If the patient is febrile, blood cultures are drawn as well as a viral screen to include respiratory viruses (e.g. adenovirus, influenza A & B, parainfluenza, RSV). Blood is also taken for a Legionella complement fixation test; an estimation for pneumococcal antigen (CIE or ELISA) in blood, urine or sputum may provide a rapid diagnosis of pneumococcal infection. In chronic cor pulmonale, liver function tests reveal evidence of chronic passive congestion (elevated alkaline phosphatase and bilirubin with normal or near normal hepatic enzymes).

2. *Sputum*
   Direct inspection reveals purulent, often blood-streaked sputum. Organisms and polymorphs can be identified by gram stain. Prior antibiotic therapy, or the fastidious nature of some causative organisms (particularly Haemophilus) may prevent adequate growth on culture.

3. *Arterial blood gases*
   An arterial PaO_2 <8 kPa on air (FIO_2 0.21) defines Type I respiratory failure. Arterial hypoxaemia is caused by ventilation-perfusion mismatch, physiological shunting or hypoventilation. In hypoventilation the $PaCO_2$ is >6 kPA (so called Type II respiratory failure). Changes in the alveolar oxygen tension (PAO_2) occurring as a consequence of increases in $PaCO_2$ can be calculated from the alveolar air equation (see Ch. 5 for details). Cor pulmonale may be associated with a metabolic acidosis caused by a low cardiac output in addition to the respiratory acidosis secondary to respiratory failure.

   Profound nocturnal hypoxaemia may occur in patients with chronic obstructive bronchitis. These transient episodes of hypoxia are usually documented during rapid eye movement

(REM) sleep, and are probably responsible for cor pulmonale and secondary polycythaemia occurring in patients who have seemingly normal arterial blood gases at rest during the day. A concomitant increase in $PaCO_2$ and pulmonary artery pressure has also been documented in these patients.

4. *Chest radiograph*

   The chest radiograph may be unremarkable in cor pulmonale. In patients with emphysema there is evidence of hyperinflation, low flat diaphragms, and a reduction in pulmonary vascular markings, but these findings correlate poorly with the loss of pulmonary tissue demonstrated pathologically. The heart size is small and on the lateral radiograph the retrosternal airspace is prominent. Localised infection may be detected and bronchiectasis is typified by bronchial wall thickening and ring shadows. As the right ventricle undergoes hypertrophy and dilatation the cardiothoracic ratio increases, but neither the right atrium nor the right ventricle can be identified with certainty on the plain PA chest radiograph. Elevation in the venous pressure may cause distention of the superior vena cava and azygos vein. In severe pulmonary hypertension the proximal pulmonary arteries are prominent and there is rapid tapering of the more distal vessels and a paucity of vessels in the peripheral lung fields.

5. *Electrocardiography*

   Serial changes in the electrocardiogram in patients with chronic airflow obstruction may herald the onset of cor pulmonale. Depression of the diaphragms and an increase in the AP diameter of the chest causes the heart to rotate clockwise and to lie vertically within the chest. Other chest wall deformities (e.g. kyphoscoliosis) may make interpretation of the ECG even more difficult. In the absence of cor pulmonale these anatomical changes lead to poor anterior R wave progression, which may be confused with an antero-septal infarct. Frequently there is a vertical frontal plane P wave axis (inverted in aVL, and upright in lead III). In the presence of right ventricular hypertrophy the ECG features of pulmonary hypertension are similar to those discussed under PPH (p. 224).

6. *Pulmonary function tests*

   A detailed description of pulmonary function tests is beyond the scope of this book. The typical patient with chronic obstructive bronchitis has a reduced FEV_1, a low FEV_1/FVC ratio ($<50\%$) and an increase in airways resistance. In patients with emphysema there is evidence of air trapping, with an increase in total lung capacity (TLC), functional residual capacity (FRC), and residual volume (RV), and a low diffusing capacity (K_{co}) due to ventilation-perfusion mismatch.

7. *Echocardiography*

   Hyperventilation may make echocardiography difficult or impossible in patients with airflow obstruction because the parasternal echo 'window' is obscured by the left lung. Technically satisfactory cross-sectional images may be obtainable from the subcostal approach, in which case the changes of pulmonary hypertension are seen (see p. 224).

8. *Radionuclide studies*

   Right ventricular ejection fraction (RVEF) can be determined by the first pass or equilibrium gated techniques using ^{99m}Tc labelled autologous red cells. Resting RVEF is inversely correlated to RV 'afterload' (i.e. pulmonary artery pressure and pulmonary vascular resistance), but poorly correlated with RV end diastolic volume and RA pressure (i.e. 'preload'). In normal subjects RVEF increases with exercise but in patients with cor pulmonale it remains constant or falls; this is due to a disproportionate increase in 'afterload', rather than evidence of inherent myocardial dysfunction. Marked RV uptake of ^{201}Tl by the myocardium is more common in patients with severe pulmonary disease particularly those with RV hypertrophy and dysfunction.

   Animal studies have demonstrated left ventricular hypertrophy and abnormal compliance in pulmonary hypertension. Some patients with cor pulmonale do show abnormal LV function (in the absence of concomitant systemic hypertension or coronary artery disease) which may be related to hypoxia, acidosis, changes in 'preload', variations in intrathoracic pressure, or the inter-relationship between left and right ventricle.

9. *Cardiac catheterisation*

   Right-sided pressures may be normal at rest but increase disproportionately with mild exertion. Despite wide respiratory variations in intrathoracic pressure, the PACWP reflects LA pressure in most patients. Individual variations in RV size and geometry limit the usefulness of RV contrast angiography and this investigation does not contribute to the management of patients with cor pulmonale.

Treatment

Therapy is directed towards treating the underlying pulmonary disease, and respiratory infection. In addition, the correction of arterial hypoxaemia leads to a reduction in pulmonary vascular resistance.

Pulmonary disease

1. *Bronchodilators*

   Bronchodilators can be administered by intravenous infusion, intermittent positive pressure breathing (IPPB), nebuliser or pressurized inhaler. A combination of intravenous aminophylline and a beta$_2$ agonist (e.g. salbutamol) given by IPPB is ideal, or a nebuliser if IPPB is unavailable. As the patient improves an inhaler can be substituted or alternatively a nebuliser can be supplied for domiciliary use.

2. *Aminophylline*

   As well as a bronchodilator action, the theophyllines improve haemodynamics in patients with cor pulmonale. Both intravenous aminophylline and oral preparations (e.g. Phyllocontin) reduce pulmonary arterial pressure and left ventricular end diastolic pressure substantially. Doses of aminophylline that have little effect on airflow obstruction increase both left and right ventricular ejection fractions. PaO$_2$ is changed little by aminophylline. Side effects include nausea and vomiting, arrhythmias, and grand mal seizures.

3. *Antibiotics*

   After blood and sputum culture, the appropriate antibiotics should be administered prior to identifying the causal organism. Haemophilus influenzae and Streptococcus pneumoniae are the two most likely organisms but Klebsiella spp should also be covered. A combination of Ampicillin 1 g IV four times daily plus Gentamicin or Tobramycin 80 mg IV three times daily (with the dose adjusted according to blood levels): peak 5–12 mg/l, trough <2 mg/l is usually effective. In patients with bronchiectasis anaerobic organisms are common and can be treated with Metronidazole 500 mg eight hourly IV, high dose penicillins or chloramphenicol. Antibiotics are continued for 10–14 days depending on response. Mycoplasma infection responds to treatment with a tetracycline (e.g. Oxytetracycline 500 mg four times daily, Doxycycline 1–2 daily), and Legionella infection is treated with Erythromycin 1 g four times daily — an extended course of antibiotics (i.e. one month) is advisable for both these organisms.

4. *Corticosteroids*

   Acute exacerbations of airflow obstruction are treated with intravenous corticosteroids (hydrocortisone 200 mg four times daily), which is then switched to Prednisolone 40 or 50 mg daily in divided doses tapering over a two week period. At the time of follow-up, after the attack of cor pulmonale has been successfully treated, it may be appropriate for the patient to undergo a trial of oral steroids in the clinic with objective documentation of lung function (e.g. spirometry, peak flows, arterial blood gases) during treatment. A trial of steroids is worthwhile in any patient with severe airflow obstruction because occasional patients will show striking steroid responsiveness without any history suggestive of reversible airflow obstruction (bronchial asthma). If steroid responsiveness is documented and the condition of the patient warrants more aggressive treatment, regular use of a steroid inhaler (e.g. Becotide, Bextosol) is advised. Long-term oral steroids may become necessary, but should be considered a last resort in patients with chronic airflow obstruction.

5. *Physiotherapy*

Regular percussion assists in moving tenacious sputum and the physiotherapist also has an important role in keeping the patient awake and encouraging coughing if they are suffering from Type II respiratory failure (with CO_2 retention).

6. *Respiratory stimulants*

CNS stimulants have a place in the treatment of cor pulmonale and respiratory failure. Although respiration can be stimulated by these agents, generalised CNS stimulation and toxicity limit their use. In view of their short half-life (5–10 min), a constant infusion is preferable to intravenous bolus. Doxepram 1.5–4.0 mg/min, increased to maximum tolerance, is the drug of choice (side effects include tachycardia, systemic hypertension, dizziness, confusion and hyperactivity).

Cor pulmonale

1. *Diuretics*

Diuretics cause an immediate fall in pulmonary artery pressure by reducing circulating blood volume. Other effects include a reduction in lung water which improves blood gas exchange and oxygenation and clearing of peripheral oedema. Changes in $PaCO_2$ as a consequence of diuretic therapy are minimal. Over enthusiastic use of diuretics may lower cardiac output leading to pre-renal failure and exacerbation of fluid retention secondary to aldosterone release. Excessive diuresis is dangerous in patients with carbon dioxide retention because a hypokalaemic metabolic alkalosis can impair the sensitivity of the respiratory centre to changes in $PaCO_2$ thereby reducing ventilatory drive. Diuretic combinations (e.g. Frusemide 40 or 80 mg + Moduretic or Dyazide 1 or 2 daily) are more effective and safer than large doses of loop diuretics. Improvement in oxygenation alone may lead to a dramatic diuresis without any additional increase in medication.

2. *Oxygen*

A modest improvement in oxygenation leads to a reduction in pulmonary artery pressure, an increased diuresis, and improved cerebral function. In many patients with chronic bronchitis, ventilation is maintained by means of hypoxic drive, and in order to avoid CO_2 narcosis, supplemental oxygen should be used with extreme caution. Controlled oxygen (2–4 l/min) is administered by a Venturi mask (e.g. Ventimask) at increasing concentrations (FIO_2 0.24, 0.28, 0.30, 0.35) with frequent monitoring of the arterial blood gases. If the $PaCO_2$ shows an increasing trend >7 kPa then the FIO_2 should be reduced. A respiratory stimulant (see p. 235) may be combined with supplemental oxygen to break the vicious circle of hypoxia-pulmonary hypertension-fluid retention-hypoxia while antibiotics are being administered to treat respiratory infection.

Long-term domiciliary oxygen prevents the progressive rise in pulmonary artery pressure and pulmonary vascular resistance that occurs with time and also appears to improve long-term survival in these patients. Continuous oxygen (>18 h/day) is preferable to intermittent oxygen.

Assisted ventilation is only used as a last resort and even then it is inappropriate in most patients as considerable difficulty may be encountered in weaning the patient from the ventilator, and the prognosis in this group is very poor.

3. *Digoxin*

The major indication for digoxin is in the control of the ventricular rate in atrial fibrillation which is not infrequently associated with cor pulmonale. Experimental evidence suggests that digoxin enhances right ventricular function only when there is coexistent left ventricular disease. Digoxin may actually increase pulmonary vascular resistance and right ventricular stroke work in patients with cor pulmonale in sinus rhythm. Hypoxia, metabolic and respiratory acidosis, and hypokalaemia increase the incidence of digoxin induced side effects.

4. *Venesection*

Secondary polycythaemia causes an increase in pulmonary vascular resistance as a result of an increase in blood viscosity (see p. 229). Chronic elevation in the haematocrit (PCV >0.65) is treated by venesection but polycythaemia of this severity is uncommon in the absence of an intracardiac shunt or an abnormal circulating haemoglobin. No more than one unit of blood should be removed at any one time, and exchange with PPF or Dextran avoids circulatory collapse.

5. *Pulmonary vasodilators*

Intravenous beta$_2$ agonists (e.g. salbutamol, terbutaline, pirbuterol) not only improve airflow obstruction, but have also been shown to lower pulmonary vascular resistance and improve right ventricular function; hydrallazine also reduces pulmonary vascular resistance. Drugs having an additional action on venous capacitance vessels (e.g. nitroglycerin, nitroprusside) may have beneficial effects on right ventricular function.

16. TACHYARRHYTHMIAS

'SUPRAVENTRICULAR' ARRHYTHMIAS

1. *Sinus tachycardia*

   In an adult a resting sinus rate greater than 100/min defines sinus tachycardia. Sinus tachycardia occurs as a physiological response to exercise and emotion, and pathologically in association with anaemia, fever, hyperthyroidism, hypoxia, hypotension, myocardial dysfunction (e.g. acute myocardial infarction, dilated cardiomyopathy) and pulmonary embolism. Responds to carotid sinus massage (CSM) by gradual slowing.

2. *Atrial fibrillation*

   No detectable P waves but atrial activity in the form of fibrillation (f) waves at a frequency of 350–700/min; f waves may be coarse or fine, the latter usually indicative of long-standing atrial fibrillation. The ventricular response (R-R interval) is irregular with normal or aberrant QRS complexes. Paroxysmal atrial fibrillation eventually gives way to sustained atrial fibrillation in most cases. Atrial fibrillation may occur in association with structural heart disease, or as an isolated finding ('lone' atrial fibrillation) (Table 16.1). CSM may cause gradual slowing of the ventricular rate.

Table 16.1 Causes of atrial fibrillation

1. 'Lone' atrial fibrillation
2. Mitral valve disease
3. Hyperthyroidism
4. Ischaemic heart disease
5. Dilated cardiomyopthy (especially alcoholic)
6. Preexcitation (WPW, LGL)
7. Post cardiac surgery (CABG etc.)
8. Aortic valve disease (exclude additional MVD)
9. Congenital heart disease (e.g. ASD)
10. Pneumonia
11. Carcinoma of the bronchus
12. Pericardial constriction
13. Digoxin toxicity
14. Pulmonary embolism (uncommon)

Haemodynamic consequences of atrial fibrillation relate to the loss of atrial systole, abbreviation of ventricular diastole and associated structural heart disease.

3. *Atrial flutter*

   Usually associated with structural heart disease. Atrial rate typically 300/min (range 250 and 350/min) visible as regular flutter (F) waves best seen in V_1 or the inferior leads. A narrow QRS at a rate of 150/min is indicative of 2:1 AV block; higher grades of AV block may indicate intrinsic AV node disease or the effects of vagotonic drugs (e.g. digoxin). CSM may cause a sudden increase in the AV block (3:1, 4:1).

4. *Atrial tachycardia*

   Occurs as a result of enhanced atrial automaticity (automatic atrial tachycardia) or intra-atrial re-entry — the two mechanisms being indistinguishable on the surface ECG. P wave morphology is usually different from that seen in sinus rhythm and may be variable (multifocal atrial tachycardia). As with atrial flutter the ventricular rate is approximately 150/min due to associated 2:1 AV block. Atrial tachycardia is seen in the elderly, as a manifestation of ischaemic heart disease, pulmonary disease or digoxin toxicity. Response to CSM similar to atrial flutter.

5. *Atrioventricular nodal re-entrant tachycardia*

   An atrial or ventricular premature impulse may induce a re-entrant tachycardia in the region of the AV node either due to dissociated pathways within the AV node, an additional or split AV node, or a bypass tract with AV nodal properties; in any event the proposed mechanism is similar with a re-entry cicuit composed of a slow and a fast pathway (Fig. 16.1). The ventricular response is regular

Atria

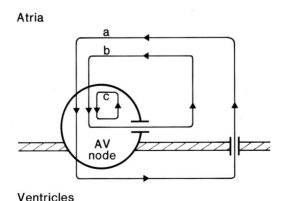

Ventricles

Fig. 16.1 Mechanism of atrioventricular nodal re-entry

(140–240/min), with a narrow QRS complex similar in morphology to that occurring in sinus rhythm. P waves may be difficult to identify because they coincide with the previous QRS. Underlying structural heart disease is uncommon. CSM and other vagal manoeuvres may convert AV nodal re-entrant tachycardia to sinus rhythm which helps differentiate it from other forms of atrial tachycardia.

6. *Atrioventricular reciprocating tachycardia*

Re-entrant tachycardia may involve an anomalous bypass tract as in the Wolff-Parkinson-White (WPW) and Lown-Ganong-Levine syndromes (LGL). These patients exhibit 'pre-excitation' and are prone to developing AV reciprocating tachycardia by a mechanism similar to that seen in AV nodal re-entrant tachycardia.

In the more common (orthodromic) form of tachycardia seen in patients with the WPW syndrome, an atrial premature beat initiates a re-entrant tachycardia that passes antegradely down the normal AV nodal pathway and retrogradely via the accessory (Kent) pathway; this results in a regular narrow complex tachycardia in which the P wave is inscribed immediately after the QRS (R-P interval < P-R interval) due to the fast retrograde conduction along the accessory pathway. Rarely the direction of the tachycardia is reversed such that antegrade conduction occurs down the accessory pathway (antidromic form); the occurrence of atrial fibrillation or flutter in this setting may be catastrophic because of the rapid ventricular response leading to a fall in cardiac output and cardiac arrest.

If the anomalous pathway is only capable of retrograde conduction, pre-excitation may be 'concealed' and the characteristic short PR interval, delta wave and broad QRS are absent on the surface ECG. In the patient with 'concealed' conduction the presence of an accessory pathway should be considered if there is history of recurrent 'supraventricular' tachycardia in an apparently fit patient, if 'supraventricular' tachycardia occurs in association with an increase in sinus rate (e.g. during exercise) or if the tachycardia has the characteristic appearance of AV reciprocating tachycardia (defined above). CSM may terminate an attack, but AV nodal re-entrant tachycardia and AV reciprocating tachycardia can only be differentiated with certainty using electrophysiological studies.

7. *Accelerated atrioventricular junctional tachycardia*

Increased automaticity of the AV node may result in an increase in the normal junctional rate (40–60/min) to a rate greater than the sinus rate (e.g. 100 min). AV dissociation may be present. This rhythm is seen in hypokalaemia, digoxin toxicity, acute myocardial infarction (usually inferior), acute myocarditis and following cardiac surgery.

VENTRICULAR ARRHYTHMIAS

1. *Ventricular tachycardia*

   Ventricular tachycardia is defined as a salvo of three or more ventricular premature beats with a rate of 100–200/min. Typical attacks may be sustained or paroxysmal and depending on the ventricular rate, features of a low cardiac output and reduced cerebral perfusion may be apparent. Ventricular tachycardia is caused by micro or macro re-entry (e.g. related to an area of infarction) or enhanced automaticity (e.g. due to electrolyte disturbance). In the majority of cases ventricular tachycardia can be differentiated from 'supraventricular' tachycardia with aberration by careful examination of the surface ECG (Table 16.2), although occasional patients require an intracardiac electrogram to determine the activation sequence with certainty.

   Ventricular tachycardia may herald ventricular fibrillation and sudden death, and in association with structural heart disease (Table 16.3) has a poor prognosis. In a minority of patients (10%) paroxysmal VT is not associated with organic heart disease in which case the prognosis is more favourable.

2. *Atypical ventricular tachycardia*

   A variety of ventricular tachycardia in which there is phasic alteration of the QRS axis (hence Torsade de pointes or

Table 16.2 ECG features of ventricular tachycardia

1. AV dissociation
2. Capture beats
3. Fusion beats
4. Blocked VA conduction
5. QRS prolongation (>140 ms)
6. Left axis deviation (QRS −30° or more)
7. Variable QRS morphology

Table 16.3 Aetiology of ventricular tachycardia

1. Ischaemic heart disease (including LV aneurysm)
2. Idiopathic dilated cardiomyopathy
3. Hypertrophic cardiomyopathy
4. Infiltrative myocardial disease (e.g. amyloid)
5. Valvular heart disease (e.g. mitral valve prolapse)
6. Drug toxicity (e.g. digoxin, catecholamines, quinidine)
7. Electrolyte imbalance (hypocalcaemia, hypokalaemia)
8. Blood gas abnormality (hypoxia)
9. Acid-base disturbance (acidosis)
10. No structural heart disease

cardiac ballet), probably due to local re-entry mechanism occurring as a result of impaired repolarisation; a number of other causes of atypical ventricular tachycardia have been recognized (Table 16.4). The unusual mechanism has important implications in the management of this arrhythmia (see p. 247). Attacks are usually self-limiting but occasionally ventricular fibrillation may ensue.

3. *Idioventricular rhythm*

   Self-terminating, usually benign arrhythmia occurring in up to 25% of patients sustaining an acute myocardial infarct; also found in digoxin toxicity and primary myocardial disease. Recognized as a regular broad complex tachycardia with a rate of 70–110/min. Mechanisms include enhanced automaticity, particularly when the basic rhythm is slow, and local re-entry initiated by a premature beat. Loss of atrial systole (as result of AV dissociation) may cause haemodynamic deterioration but this arrhythmia is usually well tolerated.

4. *Ventricular flutter*

   Highly unstable ventricular rhythm with a rate of 200–300/min characterised by a rapid sinusoidal waveform in which the QRS and ST-T waves cannot be clearly distinguished. In view of the fast rate, ventricular flutter is associated with rapid haemodynamic deterioration. Rarely recorded because ventricular flutter rapidly degenerates into ventricular fibrillation (or occasionally sinus rhythm).

5. *Ventricular fibrillation*

   Irregular and chaotic in which the waves are of variable amplitude, duration and contour due to non-uniform deplorisation and repolarisation within the ventricular myocardium. Without rapid intervention death occurs within a few minutes due to an absence of coronary and vital organ perfusion. Rarely, an episode of ventricular fibrillation may terminate spontaneously, but more commonly the coarse

---

Table 16.4 Causes of atypical ventricular tachycardia

1. Slow underlying rhythm
   (e.g. sinus bradycardia, SA block, AV block)
2. Electrolyte disturbance
   (hypokalaemia, hypomagnesaemia)
3. Long QT syndromes
   (Jervell Lange-Nielson, Romano Ward)
4. Ventricular premature beats (late)
5. Antiarrhythmic drugs
   (Classes Ia, Ib and III)
6. Psychotropic drugs
   (phenothiazines, tricyclic anti-depressants)
7. Acute myocarditis
8. Ischaemic heart disease

Table 16.5 Causes of ventricular fibrillation

1. Ischaemic heart disease
   (acute myocardial infarction, myocardial ischaemia)
2. Electrolyte disturbance (hypokalaemia)
3. Premature beats (R-on-T)
4. Pre-excitation (WPW, LGL)
5. Long QT syndromes
6. Antiarrhythmic drugs ('pro-arrhythmic effect')
7. Anaesthetic drugs (e.g. cyclopropane)
8. Sympathomimetics (e.g. adrenaline)
9. Psychotropic drugs (e.g. tricyclics)
10. Angiographic contrast media
11. DC countershock (non-synchronised)
12. Post cardiac surgery (e.g. CABG)
13. Hypothermia
14. Electrocution
15. No structural heart disease

fibrillation waves increase in rate and shorten in duration until slow bizarre complexes occur in the terminal stages prior to ventricular standstill. Most cases of ventricular fibrillation complicate acute myocardial infarction, but a mumber of other causes are known (Table 16.5).

INVESTIGATION OF ARRHYTHMIAS

1. *Physical examination*
   Character of the jugular venous pulse (e.g. presence of 'a' waves or 'cannon' waves) together with careful auscultation of the heart sounds (e.g. variation in the loudness of S1) should be part of the initial assessment of any arrhythmia and are frequently ignored.

2. *Rhythm strip*
   Fundamental to the analysis of an arrhythmia, the rhythm strip may need to be 30 seconds long to clearly identify a particular abnormality. Standard lead II or V_1 are usually chosen as they best demonstrate atrial activity. It is important to record a rhythm strip during any manoeuvre that might provoke or terminate an arrhythmia as this may give additional information as to the nature of the rhythm disturbance.

3. *Surface electrocardiogram*
   For the accurate analysis of any arrhythmia, a full 12 lead resting ECG should be recorded. Assessment of certain features (e.g. QRS axis) is not possible on a single lead rhythm strip.

4. *Carotid sinus massage*
   Firm pressure on the carotid sinus for 5–10 seconds causes an increase in vagal tone and may assist in the identification of

an arrhythmia (see individual arrhythmias for details). Each carotid should be compressed in turn as the effects of left and right CSM may differ.

5. *Holter monitor*

Ambulatory monitoring of the ECG for 24–72 hours using a portable recording device is invaluable as a means of assessing intermittent rhythm disturbances, and relating arrhythmias to symptoms experienced by the patient which are accurately recorded in a diary. Holter monitoring is also useful for assessing the response of an arrhythmia to treatment (either pharmacological or pacing), and has also been advocated as a method of documenting clinically 'silent' myocardial ischaemia by computer assisted quantification of changes in the ST segment.

6. *Exercise electrocardiogram*

Formal treadmill (or bicycle) exercise testing is usually used in the assessment of the patient with coronary artery disease (see Ch. 1). Exercise testing may also be useful as a provocative test in patients with established or possible arrhythmias. Atrial or junctional premature beats are common in normal subjects and episodes of short self-terminating atrial tachycardia are seen in 0.1–0.2% of normal studies. AV reciprocating tachycardia may be provoked in patients with pre-excitation (WPW etc.) and usually resolves spontaneously on cessation of exercise. Exercise induced ventricular premature beats are not diagnostic of coronary artery disease as they occur in 10–40% of normal subjects. Complex ectopy, sustained ventricular tachycardia, or ventricular arrhythmias occurring at a low work load are more commonly pathological, but even these are of limited prognostic value. Stress testing may also be useful in assessing the effectiveness of drug therapy in suppressing exercise induced arrhythmias.

Rate dependent bundle branch block is seen occasionally and LBBB may be mistaken for ventricular tachycardia. Patients in complete AV block should undergo stress testing prior to insertion of a dual chamber pacemaker in order to assess the atrial response to exercise (see Ch. 17).

7. *Intracardiac electrograms*

Recording the intracardiac activation sequence is a simple (and underused) method for the identification of a tachycardia, and is particularly useful in differentiating ventricular tachycardia from a 'supraventricular' tachycardia with aberrant conduction. A quadripolar electrode is inserted into the right ventricle using the standard technique for insertion of a temporary pacing electrode (see Ch. 20). Ventricular depolarisation is recorded from the distal pole, the right atrial electrogram from the proximal pole and the two displayed simultaneously with surface lead V_1 on a three channel ECG machine — thus, the activation sequence can be clearly identified.

8. *Electrophysiological study*
    Certain patients require a full intracardiac electrophysiological study in which a detailed assessment of the intracardiac activation sequence is recorded during sinus rhythm, and atrial and ventricular paced rhythm; in addition the effects of programmed stimulation and drug intervention can be analysed objectively.

TREATMENT OF ARRHYTHMIAS

General principles

Prior to treating any arrhythmia a number of questions must be asked:
1. Is the arrhythmia pathological?
2. Have all metabolic and electrolyte disturbances been corrected where possible?
3. Is pharmacological intervention the treatment of choice?
4. Is potential drug toxicity more detrimental than the arrhythmia itself?

Classification of anti-arrhythmic drugs

Vaughan-Williams classification of anti-arrhythmic drugs based on the in vitro effects of the drugs on normal cardiac cells is in common usage, and has been modified by Harrison to subdivide Class I drugs according to their effects on the duration of the action potential (Table 16.6). Difficulties may arise because certain drugs (e.g. sotalol, bretylium, amiodarone) have more than one mechanism of action in which case they are classified according to their primary action; furthermore, several important drugs (e.g. digoxin) are not included in the Vaughan-Williams classification.

In clinical practice it may be more helpful to classify the drugs according to their site of action (Table 16.7).

Table 16.6 Classification of anti-arrhythmic drugs (Vaughan-William/Harrison)

Class I: Membrane stabilising agents (inhibit fast-Na^+ channel)
  Ia: Widens QRS, prolongs QT, lengthens action potential, lengthens refractory period (e.g. quinidine, procainamide, disopyramide)
  Ib: Shortens QT, elevates fibrillation thresholds (e.g. lignocaine, mexiletine, tocainide)
  Ic: Widens QRS, little effect on duration of action potential or refractory period (e.g. flecainide, encainide, lorcainide)

Class II: Sympatholytic drugs (e.g. beta blocking agents, bretylium, bethanidine)

Class III: Drugs prolonging action potential duration (e.g. amiodarone, sotalol)

Class IV: Calcium antagonists (e.g. verapamil, diltiazem)

Table 16.7 Classification of anti-arrhythmic drugs (site of action)

Sinoatrial node	*Atria*
Class II	Class Ia, Ic
Class IV	Class II
Digoxin	Class III
Atrioventricular node	*Accessory pathways*
Class Ic	Class Ia
Class II	Class III
Class IV	
Digoxin	
	Ventricles
	Class I
	Class III

Treatment of 'supraventricular' arrhythmias

1. *Sinus tachycardia*

   Requires no specific treatment other than correcting any underlying condition.

2. *Atrial fibrillation*

   In atrial fibrillation the aim of treatment may be to restore sinus rhythm, maintain sinus rhythm or accept chronic atrial fibrillation and control the ventricular rate.

   If atrial fibrillation is recent or has been present for less than 12 months an attempt should be made to restore sinus rhythm by DC cardioversion. The risk of thromboembolism complicating DC cardioversion is approximately 1%, therefore it is advisable to anticoagulate patients with warfarin for three weeks prior to elective cardioversion if there is evidence of left atrial enlargement (by echocardiography), mitral valve disease or impaired ventricular function. A pharmacological alternative to electrical cardioversion is a disopyramide infusion. If atrial fibrillation is paroxysmal an attempt can be made to maintain sinus rhythm with oral quinidine, disopyramide or amiodarone. Anticoagulation should be continued in the groups of patients mentioned above.

   In atrial fibrillation the ventricular rate can be controlled with oral digoxin, verapamil, a beta blocker or a combination. Intravenous verapamil may be required acutely if there is haemodynamic compromise, alternatively DC countershock may be appropriate. Disopyramide or amiodarone are the drugs of choice for the treatment of atrial fibrillation occurring in a patient known to have an accessory pathway.

3. *Atrial flutter*

   Use carotid sinus massage (or other vagal manoeuvres) first. Increase AV block with digoxin together with additional verapamil or a beta blocker if necessary. Atrial fibrillation or reversion to sinus rhythm usually occurs spontaneously. As an alternative, synchronised DC countershock converts atrial flutter to sinus rhythm in more than 90% of cases. Atrial pacing may also be effective.

4. *Atrial tachycardia*

   CSM may be effective. If rapid termination is required give intravenous verapamil (or practolol); alternatively attempt DC countershock. If there is no haemodynamic compromise, load with oral digoxin.

5. *Atrioventricular nodal re-entrant tachycardia*
6. *Atrioventricular reciprocating tachycardia*

   CSM may be effective. If rapid termination required give a bolus of intravenous verapamil (practolol or disopyramide); intravenous amiodarone may also be effective. DC countershock is rarely required and casts doubt on the diagnosis. Right atrial pacing may also terminate the tachycardia. Ablative surgery is successful in certain patients. Oral disopyramide or amiodarone are suitable agents for prophylaxis against AV reciprocating tachycardia. If the arrhythmia is provoked by episodes of sinus tachycardia (e.g. on exertion) a beta blocking agent may be effective.

7. *Accelerated atrioventricular junctional tachycardia*

   Rarely requires treatment. Atropine or right atrial pacing may be effective.

Ventricular arrhythmias

1. *Ventricular tachycardia*

   For sustained ventricular tachycardia a lignocaine bolus followed by lignocaine infusion remains the treatment of choice. Flecainide, amiodarone, mexiletine, bretylium and DC countershock are also effective in abolishing ventricular tachycardia. As prophylaxis against recurrent attacks, a number of Class I (e.g. flecainide, tocainide, procainamide, disopyramide) and Class III (amiodarone, sotalol) agents are available, and the exact choice of drug may need to be determined by an electrophysiological study. Surgery may be appropriate for selected patients.

2. *Atypical ventricular tachycardia*

   Correction of metabolic and electrolyte disturbances is most important in patients with atypical ventricular tachycardia. Drugs that prolong the QT interval should be avoided (e.g. quinidine, procainamide, disopyramide, amiodarone). An attempt can be made to shorten the repolarisation time with an infusion of isoprenaline or right atrial pacing, alternatively DC countershock may be necessary.

3. *Idioventricular rhythm*

   Typical attacks are short-lived and well tolerated and require no specific treatment. Occasionally atropine will be needed to accelerate the sinus rate.

    4. *Ventricular flutter*
    5. *Ventricular fibrillation*
       Prompt DC cardioversion and cardiopulmonary resuscitation (see Ch. 20) is the treatment of choice for these malignant ventricular arrhythmias.

Specific drugs

Dose schedules are listed in Table 16.8 and pharmacokinetics in Table 16.9.

Class I: Membrane stabilising agents

Quinidine (Ia)

Prototype Class I drug still widely prescribed in the USA but rather less in the UK. Membrane stabilising agent (actions listed in Table 16.6). Due to toxicity, only the sustained action oral formulation should be used (Kinidin durules), each tablet containing quinidine bisulphate 225 mg (equivalent to quinidine sulphate BP 200 mg). Well absorbed by mouth. Commence quinidine bisulphite at a dose of 250 mg twice daily after a test dose to exclude possible hypersensitivity. Major metabolism via hydroxylation in the liver (60–90%), the remainder is excreted unchanged in the urine.

    Quinidine is one of the most effective agents for prophylaxis against atrial fibrillation, for example after successful DC cardioversion. In the UK the drug is used almost exclusively for this purpose.

    Idiosyncratic side effects limit the usefulness of quinidine. Gastrointestinal disturbance (nausea, vomiting and diarrhoea) may be particularly troublesome, in addition to the less common syndrome of cinchonism (blurred vision, headache, deafness, dizziness and vomiting). Quinidine depresses conduction and is therefore contraindicated in high grade AV block; prolongation of the QT interval may provoke atypical ventricular tachycardia. Other rare side-effects include urticaria, cardiovascular collapse, thrombocytopaenic purpura, agranulocytosis and granulomatous hepatitis (reversible).

    Quinidine interacts with digoxin to increase the plasma level, and also potentiates the effects of warfarin and possibly amiodarone.

Procainamide (Ia)

Similar effects to quinidine. Effective for atrial, junctional and ventricular tachyarrhythmias. Contraindicated in AV block, hypotension, bronchial asthma and myasthenia gravis.

    Absorption and plasma levels of oral and intravenous procainamide are similar. Active N-acetyl metabolite (NAPA) with a long half-life (6–8 h). Wide variation in blood levels after a standard dose dependent on acetylator status. In view of short half-life, sustained release preparations should be used (Procainamide Durules) sufficient to maintain the plasma concentration within the therapeutic range in divided doses.

    Most common side-effects are gastrointestinal (anorexia, bitter taste, nausea, vomiting and diarrhoea) and allergic (skin rash, pruritis, fever, agranulocytosis). Reversible drug induced lupus (not involving the kidneys) occurs in 20–70% of patients on long-term therapy.